LEADING DOCTORS ... SCIENTISTS URGE
YOU TO ...
MEDICAL NEMES...

"**Medical Nemesis** is an important book . . . There is indeed a strong case to answer."

—**The Lancet,**
journal of the British Medical Association

"An imaginative and provocative critique that identifies concerns we all share."

—Franz J. Ingelfinger, M.D.,
in **New England Journal of Medicine**

"A very important and probably indispensable book."

—Quentin D. Young, M.D.

"Disturbing and provocative . . . The urgency of the appeal and passionate commitment to radical humanism shine through."

—**New Scientist**

MEDICAL NEMESIS

The Expropriation of Health

Ivan Illich

BANTAM BOOKS
Toronto / New York / London

This low-priced Bantam Book has been completely reset in a type face designed for easy reading, and was printed from new plates. It contains the complete text of the original hard-cover edition.
NOT ONE WORD HAS BEEN OMITTED.

MEDICAL NEMESIS: THE EXPROPRIATION OF HEALTH
A Bantam Book / published by arrangement with Pantheon Books, Inc., a division of Random House, Inc.

PRINTING HISTORY
Pantheon edition published May 1976
Psychotherapy & Social Science Book Club edition published August 1976
Serializations and/or condensations appeared in EAST/WEST JOURNAL, *March 1976;* VOGUE *magazine, May 1976;* CROSS CURRENTS *magazine, May 1976,* AMERICA *magazine, May 1, 1976;* WASHINGTON POST, *May 23, 1976.*
Bantam edition / August 1977
2nd printing
3rd printing

For information address: Pantheon Books, Inc. 201 East 50th Street, New York, N.Y. 10022.

ISBN 0-553-10596-5

Bantam Books are published by Bantam Books, Inc. Its trademark, consisting of the words "Bantam Books" and the portrayal of a bantam, is registered in the United States Patent Office and in other countries. Marca Registrada. Bantam Books, Inc., 666 Fifth Avenue, New York, New York 10019.

PRINTED IN THE UNITED STATES OF AMERICA

Acknowledgments

My thinking on medical institutions was shaped over several years in periodic conversations with Roslyn Lindheim and John McKnight. Mrs. Lindheim, Professor of Architecture at the University of California at Berkeley, is shortly to publish *The Hospitalization of Space,* and John McKnight, Director of Urban Studies at Northwestern University, is working on *The Serviced Society.* Without the challenge from these two friends, I would not have found the courage to develop my last conversations with Paul Goodman into this book.

Several others have been closely connected with the growth of this text: Jean Robert and Jean P. Dupuy, who illustrated the economic thesis stated in this book with examples from time-polluting and space-distorting transportation systems; André Gorz, who has been my principal tutor in the politics of health; Marion Boyars, who with admirable competence published the draft of this book in London and thus enabled me to base my final version on a wide spectrum of critical reaction. To them and to all my critics and helpers, and especially to those who have led me to valuable reading, I owe deep gratitude.

This book would never have been written without Valentina Borremans. She has patiently assembled the documentation on which it is based, and refined my judgment and sobered my language with her constant criticism. The chapter on the industrialization of death is a summary of the notes she has assembled for her own book on the history of the face of death.

IVAN ILLICH

Cuernavaca, Mexico
January 1976

Contents

PART III. Cultural Iatrogenesis

PART IV. The Politics of Health

MEDICAL NEMESIS

The Expropriation of Health

Introduction

The medical establishment has become a major threat to health. The disabling impact of professional control over medicine has reached the proportions of an epidemic. *Iatrogenesis,* the name for this new epidemic, comes from *iatros,* the Greek word for "physician," and *genesis,* meaning "origin." Discussion of the disease of medical progress has moved up on the agendas of medical conferences, researchers concentrate on the sick-making powers of diagnosis and therapy, and reports on paradoxical damage caused by cures for sickness take up increasing space in medical dope-sheets. The health professions are on the brink of an unprecedented housecleaning campaign. "Clubs of Cos," named after the Greek Island of Doctors, have sprung up here and there, gathering physicians, glorified druggists, and their industrial sponsors as the Club of Rome has gathered "analysts" under the aegis of Ford, Fiat, and Volkswagen. Purveyors of medical services follow the example of their colleagues in other fields in adding the stick of "limits to growth" to the carrot of ever more desirable vehicles and therapies. Limits to professional health care are a rapidly growing political issue. In whose interest these limits will work will depend to a large extent on who takes the initiative in formulating the need for them: people organized for political action that challenges status-quo professional power, or the health professions intent on expanding their monopoly even further.

The public has been alerted to the perplexity and uncertainty of the best among its hygienic caretakers. The newspapers are full of reports on *volte-face* manipulations of medical leaders: the pioneers of yesterday's so-called breakthroughs warn their patients against the dangers of the miracle cures they have only just invented. Politicians who have proposed the emulation of the Russian, Swedish, or English models of socialized medicine are embarrassed that recent events show their pet systems to be highly efficient in producing the same pathogenic—that is, sickening—cures and care that capitalist medicine, albeit with less equal access, produces. A crisis of confidence in modern medicine is upon us. Merely to insist on it would be to contribute further to a self-fulfilling prophecy, and to possible panic.

This book argues that panic is out of place. Thoughtful public discussion of the iatrogenic pandemic, beginning with an insistence upon demystification of all medical matters, will not be dangerous to the commonweal. Indeed, what is dangerous is a passive public that has come to rely on superficial medical housecleanings. The crisis in medicine could allow the layman effectively to reclaim his own control over medical perception, classification, and decision-making. The laicization of the Aesculapian temple could lead to a delegitimizing of the basic religious tenets of modern medicine to which industrial societies, from the left to the right, now subscribe.

My argument is that the layman and not the physician has the potential perspective and effective power to stop the current iatrogenic epidemic. This book offers the lay reader a conceptual framework within which to assess the seamy side of progress against its more publicized benefits. It uses a model of social assessment of technological progress that I have spelled out elsewhere[1] and applied previously

[1]*Tools for Conviviality* (New York: Harper & Row, 1973).

to education[2] and transportation,[3] and that I now apply to the criticism of the professional monopoly and of the scientism in health care that prevail in all nations that have organized for high levels of industrialization. In my opinion, the sanitation of medicine is part and parcel of the socio-economic inversion with which Part IV of this book deals.

The footnotes reflect the nature of this text. I assert the right to break the monopoly that academia has exercised over all small print at the bottom of the page. Some footnotes document the information I have used to elaborate and to verify my own preconceived paradigm for optimally limited health care, a perspective that did not necessarily have any place within the mind of the person who collected the corresponding data. Occasionally, I quote my source only as an eyewitness account that is incidentally offered by the expert *author*, while refusing to accept what he says as expert *testimony* on the grounds that it is hearsay and therefore ought not to influence the relevant public decisions.

Many more footnotes provide the reader with the kind of bibliographical guidance that I would have appreciated when I first began, as an outsider, to delve into the subject of health care and tried to acquire competence in the political evaluation of medicine's effectiveness. These notes refer to library tools and reference works that I have learned to appreciate in years of single-handed exploration. They also list readings, from technical monographs to novels, that have been of use to me.

Finally, I have used the footnotes to deal with my own parenthetical, supplementary, and tangential suggestions and questions, which would have distracted the reader if kept in the main text. The layman in medicine, for whom this book is written, will himself have to acquire the competence to evaluate the

---

[2]*Deschooling Society*, Ruth N. Anshen, ed. (New York: Harper & Row, 1971).

[3]*Energy and Equity* (New York: Harper & Row, 1974).

impact of medicine on health care. Among all our contemporary experts, physicians are those trained to the highest level of specialized incompetence for this urgently needed pursuit.

The recovery from society-wide iatrogenic disease is a political task, not a professional one. It must be based on a grassroots consensus about the balance between the civil liberty to heal and the civil right to equitable health care. During the last generations the medical monopoly over health care has expanded without checks and has encroached on our liberty with regard to our own bodies. Society has transferred to physicians the exclusive right to determine what constitutes sickness, who is or might become sick, and what shall be done to such people. Deviance is now "legitimate" only when it merits and ultimately justifies medical interpretation and intervention. The social commitment to provide all citizens with almost unlimited outputs from the medical system threatens to destroy the environmental and cultural conditions needed by people to live a life of constant autonomous healing. This trend must be recognized and eventually be reversed.

Limits to medicine must be something other than professional self-limitation. I will demonstrate that the insistence of the medical guild on its unique qualifications to cure medicine itself is based on an illusion. Professional power is the result of a political delegation of autonomous authority to the health occupations which was enacted during our century by other sectors of the university-trained bourgeoisie: it cannot now be revoked by those who conceded it; it can only be delegitimized by popular agreement about the malignancy of this power. The self-medication of the medical system cannot but fail. If a public, panicked by gory revelations, were browbeaten into further support for more expert control over experts in health-care production, this would only intensify sickening care. It must now be understood that what has turned health care into a sick-making enterprise is the very intensity of an engineering endeavor that has translated human survival from the performance of organisms into the result of technical manipulation.

"Health," after all, is simply an everyday word that is used to designate the intensity with which individuals cope with their internal states and their environmental conditions. In *Homo sapiens*, "healthy" is an adjective that qualifies ethical and political actions. In part at least, the health of a population depends on the way in which political actions condition the milieu and create those circumstances that favor self-reliance, autonomy, and dignity for all, particularly the weaker. In consequence, health levels will be at their optimum when the environment brings out autonomous personal, responsible coping ability. Health levels can only decline when survival comes to depend beyond a certain point on the heteronomous (other-directed) regulation of the organism's homeostasis. Beyond a critical level of intensity, institutional health care—no matter if it takes the form of cure, prevention, or environmental engineering—is equivalent to systematic health denial.

The threat which current medicine represents to the health of populations is analogous to the threat which the volume and intensity of traffic represent to mobility, the threat which education and the media represent to learning, and the threat which urbanization represents to competence in homemaking. In each case a major institutional endeavor has turned counterproductive. Time-consuming acceleration in traffic, noisy and confusing communications, education that trains ever more people for ever higher levels of technical competence and specialized forms of generalized incompetence: these are all phenomena parallel to the production by medicine of iatrogenic disease. In each case a major institutional sector has removed society from the specific purpose for which that sector was created and technically instrumented.

Iatrogenesis cannot be understood unless it is seen as the specifically medical manifestation of *specific counterproductivity*. Specific or paradoxical counterproductivity is a negative social indicator for a diseconomy which remains locked within the system that produces it. It is a measure of the confusion delivered by the news media, the incompetence fostered by educators, or the time-loss represented by a more powerful car. Specific counterproductivity is an unwanted side-effect of increasing institutional outputs that remains internal to the system which itself originated the specific value. It is a social measure for objective frustration. This study of pathogenic medicine was undertaken in order to illustrate in the health-care field the various aspects of counterproductivity that can be observed in all major sectors of industrial society in its present stage. A similar analysis could be undertaken in other fields of industrial production, but the urgency in the field of medicine, a traditionally revered and self-congratulatory service profession, is particularly great.

Built-in iatrogenesis now affects all social relations. It is the result of internalized colonization of liberty by affluence. In rich countries medical colonization has reached sickening proportions; poor countries are quickly following suit. (The siren of one ambulance can destroy Samaritan attitudes in a whole Chilean town.) This process, which I shall call the "medicalization of life," deserves articulate political recognition. Medicine could become a prime target for political action that aims at an inversion of industrial society. Only people who have recovered the ability for mutual self-care and have learned to combine it with dependence on the application of contemporary technology will be ready to limit the industrial mode of production in other major areas as well.

A professional and physician-based health-care system that has grown beyond critical bounds is sickening for three reasons: it must produce clinical damage that outweighs its potential benefits; it cannot but enhance even as it obscures the political conditions that render society unhealthy; and it tends to mystify and to expropriate the power of the individual to heal himself and to shape his or her environment. Contemporary medical systems have outgrown these tolerable bounds. The medical and paramedical monopoly over hygienic methodology and technology is a glaring example of the political misuse of scientific achievement to strengthen industrial rather than personal growth. Such medicine is but a device to convince those who are sick and tired of society that it is they who are ill, impotent, and in need of technical repair. I will deal with these three levels of sickening medical impact in the first three parts of this book.

The balance sheet of achievement in medical technology will be drawn up in the first chapter. Many people are already apprehensive about doctors, hospitals, and the drug industry and only need data to substantiate their misgivings. Doctors already find it necessary to bolster their credibility by demanding that many treatments now common be formally outlawed. Restrictions on medical performance which professionals have come to consider mandatory are often so radical that they are not acceptable to the majority of politicians. The lack of effectiveness of costly and high-risk medicine is a now widely discussed fact from which I start, not a key issue I want to dwell on.

Part II deals with the directly health-denying effects of medicine's social organization, and Part III with the disabling impact of medical ideology on personal stamina: under three separate headings I describe the transformation of pain, impairment, and death from a personal challenge into a technical problem.

Part IV interprets health-denying medicine as typical of the counterproductivity of overindustrialized civilization and analyzes five types of political response which constitute tactically useful remedies that are all strategically futile. It distinguishes between two modes in which the person relates and adapts to his environment: autonomous (i.e., self-governing) coping and heteronomous (i.e., administered) maintenance and management. It concludes by demonstrating that only a political program aimed at the limitation of professional management of health will enable people to recover their powers for health care, and that such a program is integral to a society-wide criticism and restraint of the industrial mode of production.

Part I

Clinical Iatrogenesis

1

The Epidemics of Modern Medicine

During the past three generations the diseases afflicting Western societies have undergone dramatic changes.[1] Polio, diphtheria, and tuberculosis are vanishing; one shot of an antibiotic often cures pneumonia or syphilis; and so many mass killers have come under control that two-thirds of all deaths are now associated with the diseases of old age. Those who die young are more often than not victims of accidents, violence, or suicide.[2]

These changes in health status are generally equated with a decrease in suffering and attributed to more or to better medical care. Although almost everyone believes that at least one of his friends would

---

[1]Erwin H. Ackerknecht, *History and Geography of the Most Important Diseases* (New York: Hafner, 1965).

[2]Odin W. Anderson and Monroe Lerner, *Measuring Health Levels in the United States, 1900–1958,* Health Information Foundation Research Series no. 11 (New York: Foundation, 1960). Marc Lalonde, *A New Perspective on the Health of Canadians: A Working Document* (Ottawa: Government of Canada, April 1974). This courageous French-English report by the Canadian Federal Secretary for Health contains a multicolored centerfold documenting the change in mortality for Canada in a series of graphs.

not be alive and well except for the skill of a doctor, there is in fact no evidence of any direct relationship between this mutation of sickness and the so-called progress of medicine.[3] The changes are dependent variables of political and technological transformations, which in turn are reflected in what doctors do and say; they are not significantly related to the activities that require the preparations, status, and costly equipment in which the health professions take pride.[4] In addition, an expanding proportion of the *new* burden of disease of the last fifteen years is itself the result of medical intervention in favor of people who are or might become sick. It is doctor-made, or *iatrogenic.*[5]

---

[3]René Dubos, *The Mirage of Health: Utopian Progress and Biological Change* (New York: Anchor Books, 1959), was the first to effectively expose the delusion of producing "better health" as a dangerous and infectious medically sponsored disease. Thomas McKeown and Gordon McLachlan, eds., *Medical History and Medical Care: A Symposium of Perspectives* (New York: Oxford Univ. Press, 1971), introduce the sociology of medical pseudo-progress. John Powles, "On the Limitations of Modern Medicine," in *Science, Medicine and Man* (London: Pergamon, 1973), 1:1–30, gives a critical selection of recent English-language literature on this subject. For the U.S. situation consult Rick Carlson, *The End of Medicine* (New York: Wiley Interscience, 1975). His essay is "an empirically based brief, theoretical in nature." For his indictment of American medicine he has chosen those dimensions for which he had complete evidence of a nature he could handle. Jean-Claude Polack, *La Médecine du capital* (Paris: Maspero, 1970). A critique of the political trends that seek to endow medical technology with an effective impact on health levels by a "democratization of medical consumer products." The author discovers that these products themselves are shaped by a repressive and alienating bourgeois class structure. To use medicine for political liberation it will be necessary to "find in sickness, even when it is distorted by medical intervention, a protest against the existing social order."

[4]Daniel Greenberg, "The 'War on Cancer': Official Fiction and Harsh Facts," *Science and Government Report,* vol. 4 (December 1, 1974). This well-researched report to the layman substantiates the view that American Cancer Society proclamations that cancer is curable and progress has been made are "reminiscent of Vietnam optimism prior to the deluge."

[5]*Dorland's Illustrated Medical Dictionary,* 25th ed. (Philadelphia: Saunders, 1974): "Iatrogenic (*iatro*—Gr. physician, *gennan*—Gr. to produce). Resulting from the activity of physicians. Originally applied to disorders induced in the patient by autosuggestion based on the physician's examination, manner, or discussion, the term is

After a century of pursuit of medical utopia,[6] and contrary to current conventional wisdom,[7] medical services have not been important in producing the changes in life expectancy that have occurred. A vast amount of contemporary clinical care is incidental to the curing of disease, but the damage done by medicine to the health of individuals and populations is very significant. These facts are obvious, well documented, and well repressed.

Doctors' Effectiveness—An Illusion

The study of the evolution of disease patterns provides evidence that during the last century doctors have affected epidemics no more profoundly than did priests during earlier times. Epidemics came and went, imprecated by both but touched by neither. They are not modified any more decisively by the rituals performed in medical clinics than by those customary at religious shrines.[8] Discussion of the future of health care might usefully begin with the recognition of this fact.

The infections that prevailed at the outset of the industrial age illustrate how medicine came by its reputation.[9] Tuberculosis, for instance, reached a peak over two generations. In New York in 1812, the

---

now applied to any adverse condition in a patient occurring as the result of treatment by a physician or surgeon."

[6]Heinrich Schipperges, *Utopien der Medizin: Geschichte und Kritik der ärztlichen Ideologie des 19. Jh.* (Salzburg: Müller, 1966). A useful guide to the historical literature is Richard M. Burke, *An Historical Chronology of Tuberculosis,* 2nd ed. (Springfield, Ill.: Thomas, 1955).

[7]For an analysis of the agents and patterns that determine the epidemic spread of modern misinformation throughout a scientific community, see Derek J. de Solla Price, *Little Science, Big Science* (New York: Columbia Univ. Press, 1963).

[8]On the clerical nature of medical practice, see "Cléricalisme de la fonction médicale? Médecine et politique. Le 'Sacerdoce' médical. La Relation thérapeutique. Psychanalyse et christianisme," *Le Semeur,* suppl. 2 (1966–67).

[9]J. N. Weisfert, "Das Problem des Schwindsuchtskranken in Drama und Roman," *Deutscher Journalistenspiegel* 3 (1927): 579–82. A guide to tuberculosis as a literary motive in 19th-century drama and novel. E. Ebstein, "Die Lungenschwindsucht in der Weltliteratur," *Zeitschrift für Bücherfreunde* 5 (1913).

death rate was estimated to be higher than 700 per 10,000; by 1882, when Koch first isolated and cultured the bacillus, it had already declined to 370 per 10,000. The rate was down to 180 when the first sanatorium was opened in 1910, even though "consumption" still held second place in the mortality tables.[10] After World War II, but before antibiotics became routine, it had slipped into eleventh place with a rate of 48. Cholera,[11] dysentery,[12] and typhoid similarly peaked and dwindled outside the physician's control. By the time their etiology was understood and their therapy had become specific, these diseases had lost much of their virulence and hence their social importance. The combined death rate from scarlet fever, diphtheria, whooping cough, and measles among children up to fifteen shows that nearly 90 percent of the total decline in mortality between 1860 and 1965 had occurred before the introduction of antibiotics and widespread immunization.[13] In part this recession may be attributed to improved housing and to a decrease in the virulence of micro-organisms, but by far the most important factor was a higher host-resistance due to better nutrition. In poor countries today, diarrhea and upper-respiratory-tract infections occur more frequently, last longer, and lead to higher mortality where nutrition is poor, no matter how much or how

---

[10]René and Jean Dubos, *The White Plague: Tuberculosis, Man and Society* (Boston: Little, Brown, 1953). On the social, literary, and scientific aspects of 19th-century tuberculosis; an analysis of its incidence.

[11]Charles E. Rosenberg, *The Cholera Years: The United States in 1832, 1849, and 1866* (Chicago: Univ. of Chicago Press, 1962). The New York epidemic of 1832 was a moral dilemma from which deliverance was sought in fasting and prayer. By the time of the epidemics of 1866, the culture that had produced New York slums had as well produced chloride of lime.

[12]W. J. van Zijl, "Studies on Diarrheal Disease in Seven Countries," *Bulletin of the World Health Organization* 35 (1966): 249–61. Reduction in diarrheal diseases is brought about by a better water supply and sanitation, never by curative intervention.

[13]R. R. Porter, *The Contribution of the Biological and Medical Sciences to Human Welfare,* Presidential Address to the British Association for the Advancement of Science, Swansea Meeting, 1971 (London: the Association, 1972), p. 95.

little medical care is available.[14] In England, by the middle of the nineteenth century, infectious epidemics had been replaced by major malnutrition syndromes, such as rickets and pellagra. These in turn peaked and vanished, to be replaced by the diseases of early childhood and, somewhat later, by an increase in duodenal ulcers in young men. When these declined, the modern epidemics took over: coronary heart disease, emphysema, bronchitis, obesity, hypertension, cancer (especially of the lungs), arthritis, diabetes, and so-called mental disorders. Despite intensive research, we have no complete explanation for the genesis of these changes.[15] But two things are certain: the professional practice of physicians cannot be credited with the elimination of old forms of mortality or morbidity, nor should it be blamed for the increased expectancy of life spent in suffering from the new diseases. For more than a century, analysis of disease trends has shown that the environment is the primary determinant of the state of general health of any population.[16] Medical geography,[17] the

---

[14]N. S. Scrimshaw, C. E. Taylor, and John E. Gordon, *Interactions of Nutrition and Infection* (Geneva: World Health Organization, 1968).

[15]John Cassel, "Physical Illness in Response to Stress," Antología A7, mimeographed (Cuernavaca: CIDOC [Centro Intercultural de Documentación], 1971).

[16]One of the clearest statements on the paramount importance of the environment is J. P. Frank, *Akademische Rede vom Volkselend als der Mutter der Krankheiten* (Pavia, 1790; reprint ed., Leipzig: Barth, 1960). Thomas McKeown and R. G. Record, "Reasons for the Decline in Mortality in England and Wales During the Nineteenth Century," *Population Studies* 16 (1962): 94–122. Edwin Chadwick, *Report on the Sanitary Condition of the Labouring Population of Great Britain, 1842,* ed. M. W. Flinn (Chicago: Aldine, 1965), concluded a century and a half ago that "the primary and most important measures and at the same time the most practical, and within the recognized providence of public administration, are drainage, the removal of all refuse from habitations, streets, and roads, and the improvement of the supplies of water." Max von Petterkofer, *The Value of Health to a City: Two Lectures Delivered in 1873,* trans. Henry E. Sigerist (Baltimore: Johns Hopkins, 1941), calculated a century ago the cost of health to the city of Munich in terms of average wages lost and medical costs created. Public services, especially better water and sewage disposal, he argued, would lower the death rate, morbidity, and absenteeism and this would

history of diseases,[18] medical anthropology,[19] and the social history of attitudes towards illness[20] have shown that food,[21] water,[22] and air,[23] in correlation

---

pay for itself. Epidemiological research has entirely confirmed these humanistic convictions: Delpit-Morando, Radenac, and Vilain, *Disparités régionales en matière de santé,* Bulletin de Statistique du Ministère de la Santé et de la Sécurité Sociale No. 3, 1973; Warren Winkelstein, Jr., "Epidemiological Considerations Underlying the Allocation of Health and Disease Care Resources," *International Journal of Epidemiology* 1, no. 1 (1972): 69–74; F. Fagnani, *Santé, consommation médicale et environnement: Problèmes et méthodes* (Paris: Mouton, 1973).

[17]N. D. McGlashan, ed., *Medical Geography: Techniques and Field Studies* (New York: Barnes & Noble, 1973). Jacques May and Donna McLelland, eds., *Studies in Medical Geography,* 10 vols. (New York: Hafner, 1961–71). Daniel Noin, *La Géographie démographique de la France* (Paris: PUF, 1973). J. Vallin, *La Mortalité en France par tranches depuis 1899* (Paris: PUF, 1973). L. D. Stamp, *The Geography of Life and Death* (Ithaca, N.Y.: Cornell Univ. Press, 1965). E. Rodenwaldt et al., *Weltseuchenatlas* (Hamburg, 1956). John Melton Hunter, *The Geography of Health and Disease,* Studies in Geography no. 6 (Chapel Hill: Univ. of North Carolina Press, 1974).

[18]Erwin H. Ackerknecht, *Therapeutics: From the Primitives to the Twentieth Century* (New York: Hafner, 1973). A simple overview. J. F. D. Shrewsbury, *A History of the Bubonic Plague in the British Isles* (Cambridge: Cambridge Univ. Press, 1970). An outstanding example of history written by a bacteriologist and epidemiologist.

[19]For an introduction to the literature, see Steven Polgar, "Health and Human Behaviour: Areas of Interest Common to the Social and Medical Sciences," *Current Anthropology* 3 (April 1962): 159–205. Polgar gives a critical evaluation of each item and the responses of a large number of colleagues to his evaluation. See also Steven Polgar, "Health," in *International Encyclopedia of the Social Sciences* (1968), 6:330–6; Eliot Freidson, "The Sociology of Medicine: A Trend Report and Bibliography," *Current Sociology,* 1961–62, nos. 10–11, pp. 123–92.

[20]Paul Slack, "Disease and the Social Historian," *Times Literary Supplement,* March 8, 1974, pp. 233–4. A critical review article. Catherine Rollet and Agnès Souriac, "Épidémies et mentalités: Le Choléra de 1832 en Seine-et-Oise," *Annales Économies, Sociétés, Civilisations,* 1974, no. 4, pp. 935–65.

[21]Alan Berg, *The Nutrition Factor: Its Role in National Development* (Washington, D.C.: Brookings Institution, 1973). Hans J. Teuteberg and Günter Wiegelmann. *Der Wandel der Nahrungsgewohnheiten unter dem Einfluss der Industrialisierung* (Göttingen: Vandenhoeck & Ruprecht, 1972), deal with the impact of industrialization on the quantity, quality, and distribution of food in 19th-century Europe. With the transition from subsistence on limited staples to either managed or chosen menus, the traditional regional cultures of eating, fasting, and surviving hunger were destroyed. A

with the level of sociopolitical equality[24] and the cultural mechanisms that make it possible to keep

---

badly organized rich mine of bibliographic information. In the wake of Marc Bloch and Lucien Febvre, some of the most valuable research on the significance of food to power structures and health levels was done. For an orientation on the method used, consult Guy Thuillier, "Note sur les sources de l'histoire régionale de l'alimentation au XIXe siècle," *Annales Économies, Sociétés, Civilisations,* 1968, no. 6, pp. 1301–19; Guy Thuillier, "Au XIXe siècle: L'Alimentation en Nivernais," *Annales,* 1965, no. 6, pp. 1163–84. For a masterpiece consult François Lebrun, *Les Hommes et la mort en Anjou au 17e et 18e siècles: Essai de démographie et psychologie historiques* (Paris: Mouton, 1971); A. Poitrineau, "L'Alimentation populaire en Auvergne au XVIIIe siècle," in *Enquêtes,* pp. 323–31. Owsei Temkin, *Nutrition from Classical Antiquity to the Baroque,* Human Nutrition Monograph 3, New York, 1962. For the transformation of bread into a substance machines can produce, see Siegfried Giedion, *Mechanization Takes Command: A Contribution to Anonymous History* (New York: Norton, 1969), especially pts. 4:2, 4:3 (on meat). Also Fernand Braudel, "Le Superflu et l'ordinaire: Nourriture et boissons," in *Civilisation matérielle et capitalisme* (Paris: Colin, 1967), pp. 134–98.

[22]I. D. Carruthers, *Impact and Economics of Community Water Supply: A Study of Rural Water Investment in Kenya,* Wye College, Ashford, Kent, 1973; on the impact of water supply on health. On the improvement of rural water supplies during the 19th century: Guy Thuillier, "Pour une histoire régionale de l'eau en Nivernais au XIXe siècle," *Annales Économies, Sociétés, Civilisations,* 1968, no. 1, pp. 49 ff. The improvement of water supplies changed people's attitude towards their own bodies: Guy Thuillier, "Pour une histoire de l'hygiène corporelle. Un exemple régional: le Nivernais," *Revue d'histoire économique et sociale* 46, no. 2 (1968): 232–53; Lawrence Wright, *Clean and Decent: The Fascinating History of the Bathroom and the Water Closet and of Sundry Habits, Fashions and Accessories of the Toilet, Principally in Great Britain, France and America* (Toronto: Univ. of Toronto Press, 1967). New patterns for laundry developed: Guy Thuillier, "Pour une histoire de la lessive au XIXe siècle," *Annales,* 1969, no. 2, pp. 355–90.

[23]Lester B. Lave and Eugene P. Seskin, "Air Pollution and Human Health," *Science* 169 (1970): 723–33. Jean-Paul Dessaive et al., *Médecins, climat et épidémies à la fin du XVIIIe siècle* (Paris: Mouton, 1972).

[24]A synthetic, well-documented argument to this point is Emanuel de Kadt, "Inequality and Health," Univ. of Sussex, January 1975. The original and longer version of this paper was written in 1972 as the introductory chapter of a book, *Salud y bienestar,* which should have been published in Santiago, Chile, in 1973. John Powles, "Health and Industrialisation in Britain: The Interaction of Substantive and Ideological Change," prepared for a Colloquium on the Adaptability of Man to Urban Life, First World Congress on Environmental Medicine and Biology, Paris, July 1–5, 1974. C. Ferrero, "Health and Levels of Living in Latin America," *Milbank Memorial Fund*

the population stable,[25] play the decisive role in determining how healthy grown-ups feel and at what age adults tend to die. As the older causes of disease recede, a new kind of malnutrition is becoming the most rapidly expanding modern epidemic.[26] One-

---

Quarterly 43 (October 1965): 281–95. A decline in mortality is not to be anticipated from more expenditures on health care but from a different allocation of funds within the health sector combined with social change.

[25]Emily R. Coleman, "L'Infanticide dans le haut moyen âge," trans. A. Chamoux, *Annales Économies, Sociétés, Civilisations,* 1974, no. 2, pp. 315–35. Suggests that infanticide in the Middle Ages was demographically significant. Ansley J. Coale, "The Decline of Fertility in Europe from the French Revolution to World War II," in S. J. Behrman et al., *Fertility and Family Planning* (Ann Arbor: Univ. of Michigan Press, 1970). Marital fertility declined everywhere before the proportion of the population who married increased. Discrimination against the illegitimate combined with restricted access to marriage may have served to control population. This hypothesis is reinforced in J.-L. Flandrin, "Contraception, mariage et relations amoureuses dans l'Occident chrétien," *Annales,* 1969, no. 6 pp. 1370–90. Demographic data suggest no contraception within marriage for 17th and 18th-century France, but very low rates of illegitimacy. Contraception in marriage was near heresy, conception outside marriage a scandal. Flandrin suggests that during the 19th century sexual behavior between spouses began to be modeled on traditional behavior outside marriage. Contraception seems to have become acceptable first among peasant families rich enough to keep infant mortality low: see M. Leridon, "Fécondité et mortalité infantile dans trois villages bavarois: Une Analyse de données individualisées du XIXe siècle," *Population* 5 (1969): 997–1002. Although physicians in England opposed its spread, they seemingly applied it effectively in their own lives: J. A. Banks, "Family Planning and Birth Control in Victorian Times," paper read at the Second Annual Conference, of the Society for the History of Medicine, Leicester Univ., 1972. The Catholic Church seems to have made contraception an issue only insofar as it affected the industrial middle classes: see John Thomas Noonan, *Contraception: A History of Its Treatment by the Catholic Theologians and Canonists* (Cambridge: Harvard Univ. Press, 1965). Philippe Ariès, "Les Techniques de la mort," in *Histoire des populations françaises et de leurs attitudes devant la vie depuis le XVIIIe siècle* (Paris: Seuil, 1971), p. 373.

[26]So far, world hunger and world malnutrition have increased with industrial development. "One third to one half of humanity are said to be going to bed hungry every night. In the Stone Age the fraction must have been smaller. This is the era of unprecedented hunger. Now, in the time of the greatest technical power, starvation is an institution." Marshall Sahlins, *Stone Age Economics* (Chicago: Aldine, 1972), p. 23.

third of humanity survives on a level of undernourishment which would formerly have been lethal, while more and more rich people absorb ever greater amounts of poisons and mutagens in their food.[27]

Some modern techniques, often developed with the help of doctors, and optimally effective when they become part of the culture and environment or when they are applied independently of professional delivery, have also effected changes in general health, but to a lesser degree. Among these can be included contraception, smallpox vaccination of infants, and such nonmedical health measures as the treatment of water and sewage, the use of soap and scissors by midwives, and some antibacterial and insecticidal procedures. The importance of many of these practices was first recognized and stated by doctors—often courageous dissidents who suffered for their recommendations[28] —but this does not consign soap, pincers, vaccination needles, delousing preparations, or condoms to the category of "medical equipment." The most recent shifts in mortality from younger to older groups can be explained by the incorporation of these procedures and devices into the layman's culture.

In contrast to environmental improvements and modern nonprofessional health measures, the specifically medical treatment of people is never signifi-

---

[27] J. E. Davies and W. F. Edmundson, *Epidemiology of DDT* (Mount Kisco, N.Y.: Future, 1972). A good example of paradoxical disease control from Borneo: Insecticides used in villages to control malaria vectors also accumulated in cockroaches, most of which are resistant. Geckoes fed on these, became lethargic, and fell prey to cats. The cats died, rats multiplied, and with rats came the threat of epidemic bubonic plague. The army had to parachute cats into the jungle village (*Conservation News,* July 1973).

[28] A good example of medical persecution of innovators is given by G. Gortvay and I. Zoltan, *I. Semmelweis, His Life and Work* (Budapest: Akademiai Kiado, 1968), a critical biography of the first gynecologist to use antiseptic procedures in his wards. In 1848 he reduced mortality from puerperal fever by a factor of 15 and was thereupon dismissed and ostracized by his colleagues, who were offended at the idea that physicians could be carriers of death. Morton Thompson's novel *The Cry and the Covenant* (New York: New American Library, 1973) makes Semmelweis come alive.

cantly related to a decline in the compound disease burden or to a rise in life expectancy.[29] Neither the proportion of doctors in a population nor the clinical tools at their disposal nor the number of hospital beds is a causal factor in the striking changes in overall patterns of disease. The new techniques for recognizing and treating such conditions as pernicious anemia and hypertension, or for correcting congenital malformations by surgical intervention, redefine but do not reduce morbidity. The fact that the doctor population is higher where certain diseases have become rare has little to do with the doctors' ability to control or eliminate them.[30] It simply means that doctors deploy themselves as they like, more so than other professionals, and that they tend to gather where the climate is healthy, where the water is clean, and where people are employed and can pay for their services.[31]

---

[29]Charles T. Stewart, Jr., "Allocation of Resources to Health," *Journal of Human Resources* 6, no. 1 (1971): 103–21. Stewart classifies resources devoted to health as treatment, prevention, information, and research. In all nations of the Western Hemisphere, prevention (e.g., potable water) and education are significantly related to life expectancy, but none of the "treatment variables" are so related.

[30]Reuel A. Stallones, in *Environment, Ecology, and Epidemiology*, Pan-American Health Organization Scientific Publication no. 231 (Washington, September 30, 1971), shows there is a strong positive correlation in the U.S.A. between a high proportion of doctors in the general population and a high rate of coronary disease, while the correlation is strongly negative for cerebral vascular disease. Stallones points out that this says nothing about a possible influence of doctors on either. Morbidity and mortality are an integral part of the human environment and unrelated to the efforts made to control any specific disease.

[31]Alain Letourmy and François Gibert, *Santé, environnement, consommations médicales: Un Modèle et son estimation à partir des données de mortalité; Rapport principal* (Paris: CÉRÈBE (Centre de Recherche sur le Bien-être), June 1974). Compares mortality rates in different regions of France; they are unrelated to medical density, highly related to the fat content of the sauces typical of each region, and somewhat less to alcohol consumption.

Useless Medical Treatment

Awe-inspiring medical technology has combined with egalitarian rhetoric to create the impression that contemporary medicine is highly effective. Undoubtedly, during the last generation, a limited number of specific procedures have become extremely useful. But where they are not monopolized by professionals as tools of their trade, those which are applicable to widespread diseases are usually very inexpensive and require a minimum of personal skills, materials, and custodial services from hospitals. In contrast, most of today's skyrocketing medical expenditures are destined for the kind of diagnosis and treatment whose effectiveness at best is doubtful.[32] To make this point I will distinguish between infectious and noninfectious diseases.

In the case of infectious diseases, chemotherapy has played a significant role in the control of pneumonia, gonorrhea, and syphilis. Death from pneumonia, once the "old man's friend," declined yearly by 5 to 8 percent after sulphonamides and antibiotics came on the market. Syphilis, yaws, and many cases of malaria and typhoid can be cured quickly and easily. The rising rate of venereal disease is due to new mores, not to ineffectual medicine. The reappearance of malaria is due to the development of pesticide-resistant mosquitoes and not to any lack of new antimalarial drugs.[33] Immunization has almost wiped out paralytic poliomyelitis, a disease of de-

---

[32]The model study on this matter at present seems to be A. L. Cochrane, *Effectiveness and Efficiency: Random Reflections on Health Services*, Nuffield Provincial Hospitals Trust, 1972. See also *British Medical Journal*, 1974, 4:5. A. Querido, *Efficiency of Medical Care* (New York: International Publications, 1963).

[33]Jacques M. May, "Influence of Environmental Transformation in Changing the Map of Disease," in M. Taghi Farvar and John P. Milton, eds., *The Careless Technology* (Garden City, N.Y.: Natural History Press, 1972), pp. 19–34. May warns that mosquito resistance to insecticides on the one hand and parasite resistance to chemotherapeutic agents on the other may have created an unanswerable challenge to human adaptation.

veloped countries, and vaccines have certainly contributed to the decline of whooping cough and measles,[34] thus seeming to confirm the popular belief in "medical progress."[35] But for most other infections, medicine can show no comparable results. Drug treatment has helped to reduce mortality from tuberculosis, tetanus, diphtheria, and scarlet fever, but in the total decline of mortality or morbidity from these diseases, chemotherapy played a minor and possibly insignificant role.[36] Malaria, leishmaniasis, and sleeping sickness indeed receded for a time under the onslaught of chemical attack, but are now on the rise again.[37]

The effectiveness of medical intervention in combating noninfectious diseases is even more questionable. In some situations and for some conditions, effective progress has indeed been demonstrated: the partial prevention of caries through fluoridation of water is possible, though at a cost not fully under-

---

[34]Henry J. Parish, *A History of Immunization* (Edinburgh: Livingstone, 1965). Consult historical introduction for literature. The effectiveness of prevention in relation to any specific disease must be distinguished from its contribution to the volume of disease: J. H. Alston, *A New Look at Infectious Disease* (London: Pitman, 1967), shows how infections are replaced by new ones, without reduction in over-all volume. Keith Mellanby, *Pesticides and Pollution* (New York: Collins, 1967), in an easily understandable way demonstrates how the engineering mechanisms designed to reduce one infection foster others.

[35]República de Cuba, Ministerio de la Salud Pública, *Cuba: Organización de los servicios y nivel de salud* (Havana, 1974), introduction by Fidel Castro. An impressive demonstration of the shift in mortality and morbidity patterns over one decade during which major infections on the whole island were significantly affected by a public-health campaign. Nguyen Khac Vien, "25 Années d'activités médico-sanitaires." *Études vietnamiennes* (Hanoi), no. 25, 1970.

[36]G. O. Sofoluwe, "Promotive Medicine: A Boost to the Economy of Developing Countries," *Tropical and Geographical Medicine* 22 (June 1970): 250–4. During the 30 years between 1935 and 1968, most curative measures used for parasitic diseases and infections of the skin and respiratory organs and for diarrhea have left "the pattern of morbidity on the whole unchanged."

[37]In Farvar and Milton, eds., *The Careless Technology*, several authors make this point specifically for malaria, Bancroftian filariasis (Hamon), schistosomiasis (van der Schalie), and genito-urinary infections (Farvar).

stood.[38] Replacement therapy lessens the direct impact of diabetes, though only in the short run.[39] Through intravenous feeding, blood transfusions, and surgical techniques, more of those who get to the hospital survive trauma, but survival rates for the most common types of cancer—those which make up 90 percent of the cases—have remained virtually unchanged over the last twenty-five years. This fact has consistently been clouded by announcements from the American Cancer Society reminiscent of General Westmoreland's proclamations from Vietnam. On the other hand, the diagnostic value of the Papanicolaou vaginal smear test has been proved: if the tests are given four times a year, early intervention for cervical cancer demonstrably increases the five-year survival rate. Some skin-cancer treatment is highly effective. But there is little evidence of effective treatment of most other cancers.[40] The five-year survival rate in breast-cancer cases is 50 percent, regardless of the frequency of medical check-ups and

---

[38]Bruce Mitchel, *Fluoridation Bibliography*, Council of Planning Librarians Exchange Bibliography no. 268 (Waterloo, Ont., March 1972). Covers the debate and especially the social scientist's perception of people's behavior regarding fluoridation in Canada.

[39]C. L. Meinert et al., "A Study of the Effects of Hypoglycemic Agents on Vascular Complications in Patients with Adult-Onset Diabetes. II. Mortality Results, 1970," *Diabetes* 19, suppl. 2 (1970): 789–830. G. L. Knatterud et al., "Effects of Hypoglycemic Agents on Vascular Complications in Patients with Adult-Onset Diabetes," *Journal of the American Medical Association* 217 (1971): 777–84. Cochrane, *Effectiveness and Efficiency*, comments on the last two. They suggest that giving tolbutamide and phenformin is definitely disadvantageous in the treatment of mature diabetics and that there is no advantage in giving insulin rather than a diet.

[40]H. Oeser, *Krebsbekämpfung: Hoffnung und Realität* (Stuttgart: Thieme, 1974). This is so far, to my knowledge, the most useful introduction for the general physician or layman to a critical evaluation of world literature on the effectiveness of cancer treatment. See also N. E. McKinnon, "The Effects of Control Programs on Cancer Mortality," *Canadian Medical Association Journal* 82 (1960): 1308–12. K. T. Evans, "Breast Cancer Symposium: Points in the Practical Management of Breast Cancer. Are Physical Methods of Diagnosis of Value?" *British Journal of Surgery* 56 (1969): 784–6. Bailar, John C., "Mammography: a contrary view." in: Annals of Internal Medicine, Vol. 84, No. 1, January, 1976. pp 77–84. Promotion of mammography as a general public health measure is premature.

regardless of the treatment used.[41] Nor is there evidence that the rate differs from that among untreated women. Although practicing doctors and the publicists of the medical establishment stress the importance of early detection and treatment of this and several other types of cancer, epidemiologists have begun to doubt that early intervention can alter the rate of survival.[42] Surgery and chemotherapy for rare congenital and rheumatic heart disease have increased the chances for an active life for some of those who suffer from degenerative conditions.[43] The medical treatment of common cardiovascular disease[44]

---

[41]Edwin F. Lewison, "An Appraisal of Long-Term Results in Surgical Treatment of Breast Cancer," *Journal of the American Medical Association* 186 (1963): 975–8. "The most impressive feature of the surgical treatment of breast cancer is the striking similarity and surprising uniformity of long-term end results despite widely differing therapeutic techniques as reported from this country and abroad." The same can be said today. Constanza, Mary E., "Sounding board. The problem of breast cancer prophylaxis." in: *The New England Journal of Medicine,* Vol. 293, No. 21, Nov. 20, 1975. pp 1095–1098.

[42]Robert Sutherland, *Cancer: The Significance of Delay* (London: Butterworth, 1960), pp. 196–202. Also Hedley Atkins et al., "Treatment of Early Breast Cancer: A Report after Ten Years of Clinical Trial," *British Medical Journal,* 1972, 2:423–9; also p. 417. D. P. Byar and Veterans Administration Cooperative Urological Research Group, "Survival of Patients with Incidentally Found Microscopic Cancer of the Prostate: Result of Clinical Trial of Conservative Treatment," *Journal of Urology* 108 (December 1972): 908–13. Random comparison of four treatments (placebo, estrogen, placebo and orchiectomy, and estrogen and orchiectomy) reveals no significant differences among them, nor in comparison with radical prostatectomy. For a broad survey of analogous research on cancer in various sites, see note 40 above.

[43]Ann G. Kutner, "Current Status of Steroid Therapy in Rheumatic Fever," *American Heart Journal* 70 (August 1965): 147–9. Rheumatic Fever Working Party of the Medical Research Council of Great Britain and Subcommittee of Principal Investigators of the American Council on Rheumatic Fever and Congenital Heart Disease, American Heart Association, "Treatment of Acute Rheumatic Fever in Children: A Cooperative Clinical Trial of ACTH, Cortisone and Aspirin," *British Medical Journal,* 1955, 1:555–74.

[44]Albert N. Brest, "Treatment of Coronary Occlusive Disease: Critical Review," *Diseases of the Chest* 45 (January 1964): 40–45. Malcolm I. Lindsay and Ralph E. Spiekerman, "Re-evaluation of Therapy of Acute Myocardial Infarction," *American Heart Journal* 67 (April 1964): 559–64. Harvey D. Cain et al., "Current Therapy of Cardiovascular Disease," *Geriatrics* 18 (July 1963): 507–18.

and the intensive treatment of heart disease,[45] however, are effective only when rather exceptional circumstances combine that are outside the physician's control. The drug treatment of high blood pressure is effective and warrants the risk of side-effects in the few in whom it is a malignant condition; it represents a considerable risk of serious harm, far outweighing any proven benefit, for the 10 to 20 million Americans on whom rash artery-plumbers are trying to foist it.[46]

Doctor-Inflicted Injuries

Unfortunately, futile but otherwise harmless medical care is the least important of the damages a proliferating medical enterprise inflicts on contemporary society. The pain, dysfunction, disability, and anguish resulting from technical medical intervention now rival the morbidity due to traffic and industrial accidents and even war-related activities, and make the impact of medicine one of the most rapidly spreading epidemics of our time. Among murderous institutional torts, only modern malnutrition injures more people than iatrogenic disease in its various manifestations.[47] In the most narrow sense, iatrogenic disease includes only illnesses that would not have come about if sound and professionally recom-

---

[45] H. G. Mather et al., "Acute Myocardial Infarction: Home and Hospital Treatment," *British Medical Journal*, 1971, 3:334–8.

[46] Combined Staff Clinic, "Recent Advances in Hypertension," *American Journal of Medicine* 39 (October 1965): 634–8.

[47] Literally "iatro-genic" means an action that produces physicians, i.e. something that only medical schools or parents of future doctors do. But for over 80 years the term has been commonly used for health-damage induced by doctors. For some of the standard textbooks see Robert H. Moser, *The Disease of Medical Progress: A Study of Iatrogenic Disease*, 3rd ed. (Springfield, Ill.: Thomas, 1969). David M. Spain, *The Complications of Modern Medical Practices* (New York: Grune & Stratton, 1963). H. P. Kümmerle and N. Goossens, *Klinik und Therapie der Nebenwirkungen* (Stuttgart: Thieme, 1973 [1st ed., 1960]). R. Heintz, *Erkrankungen durch Arzneimittel: Diagnostik, Klinik, Pathogenese, Therapie* (Stuttgart: Thieme, 1966). Guy Duchesnay, *Le Risque thérapeutique* (Paris: Doin, 1954). P. F. D'Arcy and J. P. Griffin, *Iatrogenic Disease* (New York: Oxford Univ. Press, 1972).

mended treatment had *not* been applied.[48] Within this definition, a patient could sue his therapist if the latter, in the course of his management, failed to apply a recommended treatment that, in the physician's opinion, would have risked making him sick. In a more general and more widely accepted sense, clinical iatrogenic disease comprises all clinical conditions for which remedies, physicians, or hospitals are the pathogens, or "sickening" agents. I will call this plethora of therapeutic side-effects *clinical iatrogenesis.* They are as old as medicine itself,[49] and have always been a subject of medical studies.[50]

Medicines have always been potentially poisonous, but their unwanted side-effects have increased with their power[51] and widespread use.[52] Every

---

[48]For the evolution of jurisprudence related to this kind of torts see M. N. Zald, "The Social Control of General Hospitals," in B. S. Georgopoulos, ed., *Organization Research on Health Institutions* (Ann Arbor: Univ. of Michigan, Institute for Social Research, 1972). See also Angela Holder, *Medical Malpractice Law* (New York: Wiley, 1974).

[49]Such side-effects were studied by the Arabs. Al-Razi (A.D. 865–925), the medical chief of the hospital of Baghdad, was concerned with the medical study of iatrogenesis, according to Al-Nadim in the *Fihrist,* chap. 7 sec. 3. At the time of Al-Nadim (A.D. 935), three books and one letter of Al-Razi on the subject were still available: *The Mistakes in the Purpose of Physicians; On Purging Fever Patients Before the Time Is Ripe; The Reason Why the Ignorant Physicians, the Common People, and the Women in Cities Are More Successful Than Men of Science in Treating Certain Diseases and the Excuses Which Physicians Make for This;* and the letter: "Why a Clever Physician Does Not Have the Power to Heal All Diseases, for That Is Not Within the Realm of the Possible."

[50]See also Erwin H. Ackerknecht, "Zur Geschichte der iatrogenen Krankheiten," *Gesnerus* 27 (1970): 57–63. He distinguishes three waves, or periods, since 1750 when the study of iatrogenesis was considered important by the medical establishment. Erwin H. Ackerknecht, "Zur Geschichte der iatrogenen Erkrankungen des Nervensystems," *Therapeutische Umschau/Revue thérapeutique* 27, no. 6 (1970): 345–6. A short survey of medical awareness of the side-effects of drugs on the central nervous system, starting with Avicenna (980–1037) on mercury.

[51]L. Meyler, *Side Effects of Drugs* (Baltimore: Williams & Wilkins, 1972). *Adverse Reactions Titles,* a monthly bibliography of titles from approximately 3,400 biomedical journals published throughout the world; published in Amsterdam since 1966. *Allergy*

twenty-four to thirty-six hours, from 50 to 80 percent of adults in the United States and the United Kingdom swallow a medically prescribed chemical. Some take the wrong drug; others get an old or a contaminated batch, and others a counterfeit;[53] others take several drugs in dangerous combinations;[54] and still others receive injections with improperly sterilized syringes.[55] Some drugs are addictive, others mutilating, and others mutagenic, although perhaps only in combination with food coloring or insecticides. In some patients, antibiotics alter the normal bacterial flora and induce a superinfection, permitting more resistant organisms to proliferate and invade the host. Other drugs contribute to the breeding of drug-resistant strains of bacteria.[56] Subtle kinds of poisoning thus have spread even faster than the bewildering variety and ubiquity of nostrums.[57] Unnecessary surgery is a

---

Information Bulletin, Allergy Information Association, Weston, Ontario.

[52]P. E. Sartwell, "Iatrogenic Disease: An Epidemiological Perspective," *International Journal of Health Services* 4 (winter 1974): 89–93.

[53]Pharmaceutical Society of Great Britain, *Identification of Drugs and Poisons* (London: the Society, 1965). Reports on drug adulteration and analysis. Margaret Kreig, *Black Market Medicine* (Englewood Cliffs, N.J.: Prentice-Hall, 1967), reports that an increasing percentage of articles sold by legitimate professional pharmacies are inert counterfeit drugs indistinguishable in packaging and presentation from the trademarked product.

[54]Morton Mintz, *By Prescription Only,* 2nd ed. (Boston: Beacon Press, 1967). (For a fuller description of this book, see below, note 98, p. 61.) Solomon Garb, *Undesirable Drug Interactions, 1974–75,* rev. ed. (New York: Springer, 1975). Includes information on inactivation, incompatibility, potentiation, and plasma binding, as well as on interference with elimination, digestion, and test procedures.

[55]B. Opitz and H. Horn, "Verhütung iatrogener Infektionen bei Schutzimpfungen," *Deutsches Gesundheitswesen* 27/24 (1972): 1131–6. On infections associated with immunization procedures.

[56]Harry N. Beaty and Robert G. Petersdorf, "Iatrogenic Factors in Infectious Disease," *Annals of Internal Medicine* 65 (October 1966): 641–56.

[57]Every year a million people—that is, 3 to 5 percent of all hospital admissions—are admitted primarily because of a negative reaction to drugs. Nicholas Wade, "Drug Regulation: FDA Replies to Charges by Economists and Industry," *Science* 179 (1973): 775–7.

standard procedure.[58] *Disabling nondiseases* result from the medical treatment of nonexistent diseases and are on the increase:[59] the number of children disabled in Massachusetts through the treatment of cardiac nondisease exceeds the number of children under effective treatment for real cardiac disease.[60]

Doctor-inflicted pain and infirmity have always been a part of medical practice.[61] Professional cal-

---

[58]Eugene Vayda, "A Comparison of Surgical Rates in Canada and in England and Wales," *New England Journal of Medicine* 289 (1973): 1224–9, shows that surgical rates in Canada in 1968 were 1.8 times greater for men and 1.6 times greater for women than in England. Discretionary operations such as tonsillectomy and adenoidectomy, hemorroidectomy, and inguinal herniorrhaphy were two or more times higher. Cholecystecomy rates were more than five times greater. The main determinants may be differences in payment of health services and available hospital beds and surgeons. Charles E. Lewis, "Variations in the Incidence of Surgery," *New England Journal of Medicine* 281 (1969): 880–4, finds three- to fourfold variations in regional rates for six common surgical procedures in the U.S.A. The number of surgeons available was found to be the significant predictor in the incidence of surgery. See also James C. Doyle, "Unnecessary Hysterectomies: Study of 6,248 Operations in Thirty-five Hospitals During 1948," *Journal of the American Medical Association* 151 (1953): 360–5. James C. Doyle, "Unnecessary Ovariectomies: Study Based on the Removal of 704 Normal Ovaries from 546 Patients," *Journal of the American Medical Association* 148 (1952): 1105–11. Thomas H. Weller, "Pediatric Perceptions: The Pediatrician and Iatric Infectious Disease," *Pediatrics* 51 (April 1973): 595–602.

[59]Clifton Meador, "The Art and Science of Nondisease," *New England Journal of Medicine* 272 (1965): 92–5. For the physician accustomed to dealing only with pathologic entities, terms such as "nondisease entity" or "nondisease" are foreign and difficult to comprehend. This paper presents, with tongue in cheek, a classification of nondisease and the important therapeutic principles based on this concept. Iatrogenic disease probably arises as often from treatment of nondisease as from treatment of disease.

[60]Abraham B. Bergman and Stanley J. Stamm, "The Morbidity of Cardiac Nondisease in School Children," *New England Journal of Medicine* 276 (1967): 1008–13. Gives one particular example from the "limbo where people either perceive themselves or are perceived by others to have a nonexistent disease. The ill effects accompanying some nondiseases are as extreme as those accompanying their counterpart diseases . . . the amount of disability from cardiac nondisease in children is estimated to be greater than that due to actual heart disease." See also J. Andriola, "A Note on Possible Iatrogenesis of Suicide," *Psychiatry* 36 (1973): 213–18.

[61]Clinical iatrogenesis has a long history. Plinius Secundus, *Naturalis Historia* 29.19: "To protect us against doctors there is no

lousness, negligence, and sheer incompetence are age-old forms of malpractice.[62] With the transformation of the doctor from an artisan exercising a skill on personally known individuals into a technician applying scientific rules to classes of patients, malpractice acquired an anonymous, almost respectable status.[63] What had formerly been considered an abuse of confidence and a moral fault can now be rationalized into the occasional breakdown of equipment and operators. In a complex technological hospital, negligence becomes "random human error" or "system breakdown," callousness becomes "scientific detachment," and incompetence becomes "a lack of

---

law against ignorance, no example of capital punishment. Doctors learn at our risk, they experiment and kill with sovereign impunity, in fact the doctor is the only one who may kill. They go further and make the patient responsible: they blame him who has succumbed." In fact, Roman law already contained some provisions against medically inflicted torts, "damnum injuria datum per medicum." Jurisprudence in Rome made the doctor legally accountable not only for ignorance and recklessness but for bumbling. A doctor who operated on a slave but did not properly follow up his convalescence had to pay the price of the slave and the loss of the master's income during his protracted sickness. Citizens were not covered by these statutes, but could avenge malpractice on their own initiative.

[62]Montesquieu, *De l'esprit des lois,* bk. 29, chap. 14, b (Paris: Pléiade, 1951). The Roman laws ordained that physicians should be punished for neglect or lack of skill (the Cornelian laws, *De Sicariis,* inst. iv. tit. 3, de lege Aquila 7). If the physician was a person of any fortune or rank, he was only condemned to deportation, but if he was of low condition he was put to death. In our institutions it is otherwise. The Roman laws were not made under the same circumstances as ours: in Rome every ignorant pretender meddled with physic, but our physicians are obliged to go through a regular course of study and to take degrees, for which reason they are supposed to understand their profession. In this passage the 17th-century philosopher demonstrates an entirely modern optimism about medical education.

[63]For German internists, the time the patient can spend face-to-face with his doctor has now been reduced to 1.7 minutes per visit. Heinrich Erdmann, Heinz-Günther Overrath, and Wolfgang and Thure Uxkull, "Organisationsprobleme der ärztlichen Krankenversorgung: Dargestellt am Beispiel einer medizinischen Universitätsklinik," *Deutsches Ärzteblatt–Ärztliche Mitteilungen* 71 (1974): 3421–6. In general practice, this time was (in 1963) about 3 minutes. See T. Geyer, *Verschwörung* (Hilchenbach: Medizinpolitischer Verlag, 1971), p. 30.

specialized equipment." The depersonalization of diagnosis and therapy has changed malpractice from an ethical into a technical problem.[64]

In 1971, between 12,000 and 15,000 malpractice suits were lodged in United States courts. Less than half of all malpractice claims were settled in less than eighteen months, and more than 10 percent of such claims remain unsettled for over six years. Between 16 and 20 percent of every dollar paid in malpractice insurance went to compensate the victim; the rest was paid to lawyers and medical experts.[65] In such cases, doctors are vulnerable only to the charge of having acted against the medical code, of the incompetent performance of prescribed treatment, or of dereliction out of greed or laziness. The problem, however, is that most of the damage inflicted by the modern doctor does not fall into any of these categories.[66] It occurs in the ordinary practice of well-trained men and women who have learned to bow to prevailing professional judgment and procedure, even though they know (or could and should know) what damage they do.

---

[64]For the broader issue of genetic rather than individual damage, see John W. Goffman and Arthur R. Tamplin, "Epidemiological Studies of Carcinogenesis by Ionizing Radiation," in *Proceedings of the Sixth Berkeley Symposium on Mathematical Statistics and Probability,* Univ. of California, July 1970, pp. 235–77. The presumption is all too common that where uncertainty exists about the magnitude of carcinogenic effects, it is appropriate to continue the exposure of humans to the risk. The authors show that it is neither appropriate nor good public-health practice to demand human epidemiological evidence before stopping exposure. The argument against ionizing radiation from nuclear generation of electrical energy can be applied to all medical treatment in which there is uncertainty about genetic impact. The competence of physicians to establish levels of tolerance for entire populations must be questioned on theoretical grounds.

[65]For data and further bibliography see U.S. House of Representatives, Committee on Interstate and Foreign Commerce, *An Overview of Medical Malpractice,* 94th Cong., 1st Sess., March 17, 1975.

[66]The maltreatment of patients has become an accepted routine; see Charles Butterworth, "Iatrogenic Malnutrition," *Nutrition Today,* March–April 1974. One of the largest pockets of unrecognized malnutrition in America and Canada exists, not in rural slums or urban ghettos, but in the private rooms and wards of big-city hospitals. J. Mayer, "Iatrogenic Malnutrition," *New England Journal of Medicine* 284 (1971): 1218.

The United States Department of Health, Education, and Welfare calculates that 7 percent of all patients suffer compensable injuries while hospitalized, though few of them do anything about it. Moreover, the frequency of reported accidents in hospitals is higher than in all industries but mines and high-rise construction. Accidents are the major cause of death in American children. In proportion to the time spent there, these accidents seem to occur more often in hospitals than in any other kind of place. One in fifty children admitted to a hospital suffers an accident which requires specific treatment.[67] University hospitals are relatively more pathogenic, or, in blunt language, more sickening. It has also been established that one out of every five patients admitted to a typical research hospital acquires an iatrogenic disease, sometimes trivial, usually requiring special treatment, and in one case in thirty leading to death. Half of these episodes result from complications of drug therapy; amazingly, one in ten comes from diagnostic procedures.[68] Despite good intentions and claims to public service, a military officer with a similar record of performance would be relieved of his command, and a restaurant or amusement center would be closed by the police. No wonder that the health industry tries to shift the blame for the damage caused onto the victim, and that the dope-sheets of a multinational pharmaceutical concern tells its readers that "iatrogenic disease is almost always of neurotic origin."[69]

Defenseless Patients

The undesirable side-effects of approved, mistaken, callous, or contraindicated technical contacts with the medical system represent just the first level of

---

[67]George H. Lowrey, "The Problem of Hospital Accidents to Children," *Pediatrics* 32 (December 1963): 1064–8.

[68]J. T. McLamb and R. R. Huntley, "The Hazards of Hospitalization," *Southern Medical Journal* 60 (May 1967): 469–72.

[69]"La maladie iatrogène est presque toujours à base névrotique": L. Israel, "La Maladie iatrogène," in *Documenta Sandoz,* n.d.

pathogenic medicine. Such *clinical iatrogenesis* includes not only the damage that doctors inflict with the intent of curing or of exploiting the patient, but also those other torts that result from the doctor's attempt to protect himself against the possibility of a suit for malpractice. Such attempts to avoid litigation and prosecution may now do more damage than any other iatrogenic stimulus.

On a second level,[70] medical practice sponsors sickness by reinforcing a morbid society that encourages people to become consumers of curative, preventive, industrial and environmental medicine. On the one hand defectives survive in increasing numbers and are fit only for life under institutional care, while on the other hand, medically certified symptoms exempt people from industrial work and thereby remove them from the scene of political struggle to reshape the society that has made them sick. Second-level iatrogenesis finds its expression in various symptoms of social overmedicalization that amounts to what I shall call the expropriation of health. This second-level impact of medicine I designate as *social iatrogenesis,* and I shall discuss it in Part II.

On a third level, the so-called health professions have an even deeper, culturally health-denying effect insofar as they destroy the potential of people to deal with their human weakness, vulnerability, and uniqueness in a personal and autonomous way. The patient in the grip of contemporary medicine is but one instance of mankind in the grip of its pernicious techniques.[71] This *cultural iatrogenesis,* which

---

[70]The distinction of several levels of iatrogenesis was made by Ralph Audy, "Man-made Maladies and Medicine," *California Medicine,* November 1970, pp. 48–53. He recognizes that iatrogenic "diseases" are only one type of man-made malady. According to their etiology, they fall into several categories: those resulting from diagnosis and treatment, those relating to social and psychological attitudes and situations, and those resulting from man-made programs for the control and eradication of disease. Besides iatrogenic clinical entities, he recognizes other maladies that have a medical etiology.

[71]"Das Schicksal des Kranken verkörpert als Symbol das Schicksal der Menschheit im Stadium einer technischen Weltentwicklung":

I shall discuss in Part III, is the ultimate backlash of hygienic progress and consists in the paralysis of healthy response to suffering, impairment, and death. It occurs when people accept health management designed on the engineering model, when they conspire in an attempt to produce, as if it were a commodity, something called "better health." This inevitably results in the managed maintenance of life on high levels of sublethal illness. This ultimate evil of medical "progress" must be clearly distinguished from both clinical and social iatrogenesis.

I hope to show that on each of its three levels iatrogenesis has become medically irreversible: a feature built right into the medical endeavor. The unwanted physiological, social, and psychological byproducts of diagnostic and therapeutic progress have become resistant to medical remedies. New devices, approaches, and organizational arrangements, which are conceived as remedies for clinical and social iatrogenesis, themselves tend to become pathogens contributing to the new epidemic. Technical and managerial measures taken on any level to avoid damaging the patient by his treatment tend to engender a self-reinforcing iatrogenic loop analogous to the escalating destruction generated by the polluting procedures used as antipollution devices.[72]

I will designate this self-reinforcing loop of negative institutional feedback by its classical Greek equivalent and call it *medical nemesis*. The Greeks saw gods in the forces of nature. For them, nemesis

---

Wolfgang Jacob, *Der kranke Mensch in der technischen Welt*, IX. Internationaler Fortbildungskurs für praktische und wissenschaftliche Pharmazie der Bundesapothekerkammer in Meran (Frankfurt am Main: Werbe- und Vertriebsgesellschaft Deutscher Apotheker, 1971).

[72]James B. Quinn, "Next Big Industry: Environmental Improvement," *Harvard Business Review* 49 (September–October 1971): 120–30. He believes that environmental improvement is becoming a dynamic and profitable series of markets for industry that pay for themselves and in the end will represent an important addition to income and GNP. Implicitly the same argument is being made for the health-care field by the proponents of no-fault malpractice insurance.

represented divine vengeance visited upon mortals who infringe on those prerogatives the gods enviously guard for themselves. Nemesis was the inevitable punishment for attempts to be a hero rather than a human being. Like most abstract Greek nouns, Nemesis took the shape of a divinity. She represented nature's response to *hubris*: to the individual's presumption in seeking to acquire the attributes of a god. Our contemporary hygienic hubris has led to the new syndrome of medical nemesis.[73]

By using the Greek term I want to emphasize that the corresponding phenomenon does not fit within the explanatory paradigm now offered by bureaucrats, therapists, and ideologues for the snowballing diseconomies and disutilities that, lacking all intuition, they have engineered and that they tend to call the "counterintuitive behavior of large systems." By invoking myths and ancestral gods I should make it clear that my framework for analysis of the current breakdown of medicine is foreign to the industrially determined logic and ethos. I believe that the *reversal of nemesis* can come only from within man and not from yet another managed (heteronomous) source depending once again on presumptuous expertise and subsequent mystification.

Medical nemesis is resistant to medical remedies. It can be reversed only through a recovery of the will to self-care among the laity, and through the legal, political, and institutional recognition of the right to care, which imposes limits upon the professional monopoly of physicians. My final chapter proposes guidelines for stemming medical nemesis and provides criteria by which the medical enterprise can be kept within healthy bounds. I do not suggest any specific forms of health care or sick-care, and I do not advocate any new medical philosophy any more than I recommend remedies for medical technique, doc-

---

[73]The term was used by Honoré Daumier (1810–79). See reproduction of his drawing "Némésis médical" in Werner Block, *Der Artzt und der Tod in Bildern aus sechs Jahrhunderten* (Stuttgart: Enke, 1966).

trine, or organization. However, I do propose an alternative approach to the use of medical organization and technology together with the allied bureaucracies and illusions.

Part II

Social Iatrogenesis

2

The Medicalization of Life

Political Transmission of Iatrogenic Disease

Until recently medicine attempted to enhance what occurs in nature. It fostered the tendency of wounds to heal, of blood to clot, and of bacteria to be overcome by natural immunity.[1] Now medicine tries to engineer the dreams of reason.[2] Oral contraceptives, for instance, are prescribed "to prevent a normal occurrence in healthy persons."[3] Therapies in-

---

[1]Judith P. Swazey and Renée Fox, "The Clinical Moratorium: A Case Study of Mitral Valve Surgery," in Paul A. Freund, ed., *Experimentation with Human Subjects* (New York: Braziller, 1970), pp. 315–57.

[2]Francisco Goya, in *Los Caprichos,* the series of etchings of 1786, shows a man asleep at his desk with his head on his crossed arms, while monsters surround him. The inscription on the desk reads, "El sueño de la razón produce monstruos." René Dubos uses this picture as frontispiece of his book *The Mirage of Health* (see above, note 3, p. 4). It encapsulates his thesis, on which I try to elaborate in the present book.

[3]Morton Mintz, *The Pill: An Alarming Report* (Boston: Beacon Press, 1970). Model for a study *of* medicine by a newspaper reporter who knows how to combine studies *in* medicine with information that is significant but has been overlooked, repressed, or veiled in medical literature.

duce the organism to interact with molecules or with machines in ways for which there is no precedent in evolution. Grafts involve the outright obliteration of genetically programmed immunological defenses.[4] The relationship between the interest of the patient and the success of each specialist who manipulates one of his "conditions" can thus no longer be assumed; it must now be proved, and the net contribution of medicine to society's burden of disease must be assessed from without the profession.[5] But any charge against medicine for the clinical damage it causes constitutes only the first step in the indictment of pathogenic medicine.[6] The trail beaten in the harvest

---

[4]Francis D. Moore, "The Therapeutic Innovation: Ethical Boundaries in the Initial Clinical Trials of New Drugs and Surgical Procedures," in Freund, ed., *Experimentation with Human Subjects,* pp. 358–78.

[5]One example of the need for such outside control over professional progress might be useful. Peter R. Breggin, "The Return of Lobotomy and Psychosurgery," *Congressional Record* 118 (February 24, 1972): 5567–77, presents a truly shocking review of the vast literature on the current resurgence of lobotomy in the U.S. and around the world. The first wave was aimed mostly (⅔) at female state hospital patients, and claimed 50,000 persons in the U.S. alone before 1964. New methods are available to destroy parts of the brain by ultrasonic waves, electric coagulation, and implantation of radium seeds. The technique is promoted for the sedation of the elderly, to render their institutionalization less expensive; for the control of hyperactive children; and to reduce erotic fantasies and the tendency to gamble.

[6]Each society has its characteristic "nosology," or classification of diseases. Both the extent of conditions classified as disease and the number and kinds of diseases listed change with history. The official or medical nosology recognized in a society can be to a very high degree out of gear with the perception of the disease shared by one or several of the society's classes. See Michel Foucault, *The Birth of the Clinic,* trans, A. M. Sheridan Smith (New York: Pantheon, 1973). In our society nosology is almost totally medicalized; ill-health that is not labeled by the physician is written off either as malingering or as illusion. As long as iatrogenic disease is treated as one small category within the established nosology, its contribution to the total volume of recognized diseases will not be appreciated. Zola, Irving Kenneth, "Medicine as an institution of social control." in: *The Sociological Review,* vol. 20 No. 4 (new series) Nov. 1972. pp. 487–509. "The theme of this essay is that medicine is becoming a major institution of social control, nudging aside, if not incorporating, the more traditional institutions of religion and law. It is becoming the new repository of truth, the place where absolute and

is only a reminder of the greater damage done by the baron to the village that his hunt overruns.

Social Iatrogenesis

Medicine undermines health not only through direct aggression against individuals but also through the impact of its social organization on the total milieu. When medical damage to individual health is produced by a sociopolitical mode of transmission, I will speak of "social iatrogenesis," a term designating all impairments to health that are due precisely to those socio-economic transformations which have been made attractive, possible, or necessary by the institutional shape health care has taken. Social iatrogenesis designates a category of etiology that encompasses many forms. It obtains when medical bureaucracy creates ill-health by increasing stress, by multiplying disabling dependence, by generating new painful needs, by lowering the levels of tolerance for discomfort or pain, by reducing the leeway that people are wont to concede to an individual when he suffers, and by abolishing even the right to self-care. Social iatrogenesis is at work when health care is turned into a standardized item, a staple; when all suffering is "hospitalized" and homes become inhospitable to birth, sickness, and death; when the language in which people could experience their bodies is turned into bureaucratic gobbledegook; or when suffering, mourning, and healing outside the patient role are labeled a form of deviance.

Medical Monopoly

Like its clinical counterpart, social iatrogenesis can escalate from an adventitious feature into an inherent characteristic of the medical system. When the

---

often final judgments are made by supposedly morally neutral and objective experts . . . in the name of health." This essay came to my attention only after I had read final proofs, and I was unable to indicate that the term "medicalization" of society in the sense in which I used it in this book had been applied to the same phenomenon in this brilliant and dense essay.

intensity[7] of biomedical intervention crosses a critical threshold, clinical iatrogenesis turns from error, accident, or fault into an incurable perversion of medical practice. In the same way, when professional autonomy degenerates into a radical monopoly[8] and people are rendered impotent to cope with their milieu, social iatrogenesis becomes the main product of the medical organization.

A radical monopoly goes deeper than that of any one corporation or any one government. It can take many forms. When cities are built around vehicles, they devalue human feet; when schools pre-empt learning, they devalue the autodidact; when hospitals draft all those who are in critical condition, they impose on society a new form of dying. Ordinary monopolies corner the market;[9] radical monopolies disable people from doing or making things on their own.[10] The commercial monopoly restricts the flow of commodities; the more insidious social monopoly paralyzes the output of nonmarketable use-values.[11] Radical monopolies impinge still further on freedom and

---

[7]I use the term "intensity" to designate an increase that can be marked by numbers but not measured directly. Paralyzing fear is by no means superior to a lesser fear that drives to flight. Fernand Renoitre, *Éléments de critique des sciences et de cosmologie,* course published by the Institut Supérieur de Philosophie, Louvain, 1947, pp. 129–30.

[8]For a more systematic analysis of the term "radical monopoly" as applied to professional institutions, see Ivan Illich, *Tools for Conviviality* (New York: Harper & Row, 1973), chap. 3, sec. 2, pp. 51–7.

[9]An example: Until about 1969, penicillin G tablets were available in Mexican pharmacies under their generic name at a very low price. They have since disappeared from the market. The *Farmacopea Mexicana* does not list any oral penicillin G even in trademark preparations. Only considerably more expensive preparations are available.

[10]John Blake, ed., *Safeguarding the Public: Historical Aspects of Medical Drug Control,* Papers from a Conference Sponsored by the National Library of Medicine (Baltimore: Johns Hopkins, 1970). On the process by which the medical profession developed its self-image of benevolent caretaker, see L. Edelstein, *The Hippocratic Oath* (Baltimore: Johns Hopkins, 1943).

[11]For the classic distinction between exchange-value and use-value consult Karl Marx, *Capital* (Chicago: Kerr, 1912), vol. 1, chap. 1, especially sec. 4.

independence. They impose a society-wide substitution of commodities for use-values by reshaping the milieu and by "appropriating" those of its general characteristics which have enabled people so far to cope on their own. Intensive education turns autodidacts into unemployables, intensive agriculture destroys the subsistence farmer, and the deployment of police undermines the community's self-control. The malignant spread of medicine has comparable results: it turns mutual care and self-medication into misdemeanors or felonies. Just as clinical iatrogenesis becomes medically incurable when it reaches a critical intensity and then can be reversed only by a decline of the enterprise, so can social iatrogenesis be reversed only by political action that retrenches professional dominance.

A radical monopoly feeds on itself. Iatrogenic medicine reinforces a morbid society in which social control of the population by the medical system turns into a principal economic activity. It serves to legitimize social arrangements into which many people do not fit. It labels the handicapped as unfit and breeds ever new categories of patients. People who are angered, sickened, and impaired by their industrial labor and leisure can escape only into a life under medical supervision and are thereby seduced or disqualified from political struggle for a healthier world.[12]

Social iatrogenesis is not yet accepted as a common etiology of disease. If it were recognized that

---

[12]Michel Bosquet, "Quand la médecine rend malade: La Terrible Accusation d'un groupe d'experts," *Le Nouvel Observateur,* no. 519 (1974), pp. 84–118, and no. 520 (1974), pp. 90–130. This article shows how social iatrogenesis is fundamentally the result of the alibi function played by the professional monopoly of the sick-role. Ernest Drucker, Victor Sidel. The communicable disease model of heroin addiction: a critique. Originally presented at the Annual Meeting of the American Public Health Assoc., Nov., 1973. Revised for publication in Sept., 1974. In: *American Journal Drug & Alcohol Abuse,* Vol. 1, No. 3, 1974. pp. 301–11. Illustrates how epidemiology is used in our society to justify many forms of sick-making corruption and to "crack down" on small groups of victims of these conditions.

diagnosis often serves as a means of turning political complaints against the stress of growth into demands for more therapies that are just more of its costly and stressful outputs, the industrial system would lose one of its major defenses.[13] At the same time, awareness of the degree to which iatrogenic ill-health is politically communicated would shake the foundations of medical power much more profoundly than any catalogue of medicine's technical faults.[14]

Value-free Cure?

The issue of social iatrogenesis is often confused with the diagnostic authority of the healer. To defuse the issue and to protect their reputation, some physicians insist on the obvious: namely, that medicine cannot be practiced without the iatrogenic creation of disease. Medicine always creates illness as a social state.[15] The recognized healer transmits to individuals the social possibilities for acting sick.[16] Each culture

---

[13]Paul Ramsey, *Fabricated Man: The Ethics of Genetic Control* (New Haven, Conn.: Yale Univ. Press, 1970), argues that there are things we can do which ought not to be done. To exclude these things is a necessary condition for safeguarding man from total abasement by technical control. Ramsey reaches this conclusion about specific kinds of medical techniques. I make the same argument, but about the global intensity of the medical endeavor.

[14]P. M. Brunetti, "Health in Ecological Perspective," *Acta Psychiatrica Scandinavica* 49, fasc. 4 (1973): 393–404. Brunetti argues that the concentration of power and the dependence on extrametabolic energy can make the vital milieu uninhabitable for beings whose integration depends on the exercise of their autonomy. Medicine is used to rationalize this transfer.

[15]Renée Fox, "Illness," in *International Encyclopedia of the Social Sciences* (1968), 7: 90–6. An excellent introduction to the evolution of this concept.

[16]Talcott Parsons, *The Social System* (New York: Free Press, 1951), pp. 428 ff., contains the classic formulation of the sick role. Miriam Siegler and Humphrey Osmond, *Models of Madness, Models of Medicine* (New York: Macmillan, forthcoming) compare several models for disabling deviance and plead, for political reasons, for the relative expansion of the Parsonian sick role on the grounds that it alone creates a claim to therapy. For the contrary plea see Niels Christie's still untitled forthcoming book on the counterproductivity of therapy. (For manuscript, write to Niels Christie, Faculty of Law and Jurisprudence, University of Oslo.)

has its own characteristic perception of disease[17] and thus its unique hygienic mask.[18] Disease takes its features from the physician who casts the actors into one of the available roles.[19] To make people legitimately sick is as implicit in the physician's power as the poisonous potential of the remedy that works.[20] The medicine man commands poisons and charms. The Greeks' only word for "drug"—*pharmakon*—did not distinguish between the power to cure and the power to kill.[21]

Medicine is a moral enterprise and therefore inevitably gives content to good and evil. In every society, medicine, like law and religion, defines what is normal, proper, or desirable. Medicine has the authority to label one man's complaint a legitimate illness, to declare a second man sick though he himself does not complain, and to refuse a third social

---

[17]Forrest E. Clements, "Primitive Concepts of Disease," *University of California Publications in American Archaeology and Ethnology* 32, no. 2 (1932): 185–252. Common etiologies fall into four main categories: (1) sorcery, (2) breach of taboo, (3) intrusion of foreign object, (4) loss of soul.

[18]Eliot Freidson, "Disability as Deviance," in M. B. Sussman, ed., *Sociology and Rehabilitation* (Washington: American Sociological Association, 1966), pp. 71–99. Professional diagnosis tends merely to give validity to lay perceptions of the value attributed to certain individuals.

[19]Harold Garfinkel, "Conditions of Successful Degradation Ceremonies," *American Journal of Sociology* 61 (March 1956): 420–44. In our society public degradation ceremonies outside the courts are rather rare. But medicine even today puts public evaluation on characteristics considered as essential as self-control or sexuality.

[20]Louis Lewin, *The Untoward Effects of Drugs,* trans. W. T. Alexandre (Detroit: Davis, 1883). Notwithstanding its early date, this remains a fascinating book to read, full of historical footnotes. It lists victims of medicine from Nero's guard captain (Spanish fly) to Otto II (aloes), and Avicenna (pepper enema).

[21]On the double meaning of this term from archaic texts to the Hippocratic corpus, see Walter Artelt, *Studien zur Geschichte der Begriffe "Heilmittel" und "Gift": Urzeit-Homer-Corpus Hippocraticum* (Darmstadt: Wissenschaftliche Buch-gesellschaft, 1968). John D. Gimlette, *Malay Poisons and Charm Cures* (Kuala Lumpur: Oxford Univ. Press, 1971); John D. Gimlette and H. W. Thompson, *A Dictionary of Malayan Medicine* (Kuala Lumpur: Oxford Univ. Press, 1971): both volumes form a fascinating introduction to the same ambiguity in an entirely different world.

recognition of his pain, his disability, and even his death.[22] It is medicine which stamps some pain as "merely subjective,"[23] some impairment as malingering,[24] and some deaths—though not others—as suicide.[25] The judge determines what is legal and who is guilty.[26] The priest declares what is holy and who has broken a taboo. The physician decides what is a symptom and who is sick. He is a moral entrepreneur,[27] charged with inquisitorial powers to discover

---

[22]Judith Lorber, "Deviance as Performance: The Case of Illness," in Eliot Freidson and Judith Lorber, eds., *Medical Men and Their Work* (Chicago: Aldine, 1972), pp. 414–23. Discusses the attempts of the deviant person to convey the impression which he hopes will lead to the imposition of a certain label rather than another.

[23]Thomas S. Szasz, "The Psychology of Persisent Pain: A Portrait of l'Homme Douloureux," in A. Soulairac, J. Cahn, and J. Charpentier, eds. *Pain,* Proceedings of the International Symposium Organized by the Laboratory of Psychophysiology, Faculty of Sciences, Paris, April 11–13, 1967 (New York: Academic Press, 1968), pp. 93–113.

[24]Mark G. Field, "Structured Strain in the Role of the Soviet Physician," *American Journal of Sociology,* 58 (1953): 493–502. Describes a situation in which the government rationed sick passes, which were in great demand by overstrained workers. Physicians were forced to readjust the definition of sickness to balance the interest of the workers against the demands of the production process. Thomas S. Szasz, "Malingering: Diagnosis or Social Condemnation?" in Freidson, and Lorber, eds., *Medical Men and Their Work,* pp. 353–68.

[25]Edwin S. Shneidman, "Orientations Towards Death: A Vital Aspect of the Study of Lives," in Robert W. White, ed., *The Study of Lives: Essays on Personality in Honor of A. Murray* (New York: Atherton, 1963). For the classification of death by intention and legitimacy and further literature on the subject, see Gregory Zilboorg, "Suicide Among Civilized and Primitive Races," *American Journal of Psychiatry* 92 (May 1936): 1347–69.

[26]Pharmacists, for instance, will not be condemned for poisoning their clients. See Earl R. Quinney, "Occupational Structure and Criminal Behavior: Prescription Violation by Retail Pharmacists," *Social Problems* 11 (1963): 179–85.

[27]Howard S. Becker, *Outsiders: Studies in the Sociology of Deviance* (New York: Free Press, 1963). Clarifies the connection between the therapeutic orientation of an occupation or profession and "entrepreneurship."

[28]Joseph R. Gusfield, "Social Structure and Moral Reform: A Study of the Woman's Christian Temperance Union," *American*

certain wrongs to be righted.[28] Medicine, like all crusades, creates a new group of outsiders each time it makes a new diagnosis stick.[29] Morality is as implicit in sickness as it is in crime or in sin.

In primitive societies it is obvious that in the exercise of medical skill, the recognition of moral power is implied. Nobody would summon the medicine man unless he conceded to him the skill of discerning evil spirits from good ones. In a higher civilization this power expands. Here medicine is exercised by full-time specialists who control large populations by means of bureaucratic institutions.[30] These specialists form professions which exercise a unique kind of control over their own work.[31] Unlike unions, these professions owe their autonomy to a grant of confidence rather than to victory in a struggle. Unlike guilds, which determine only who shall work and how, they determine also what work shall be done. In the United States the medical profession owes this supreme authority to a reform of the medical schools just before World War I. The medical profession is a manifestation in one particular sector of the control over the structure of class power which the university-trained elites have acquired. Only doctors now "know" what constitutes sickness, who is sick, and what shall be done to the sick and to those whom they consider *at a special risk.* Paradoxically, Western medicine, which has insisted on keeping its power apart from law and religion, has now expanded it beyond precedent. In some industrial societies social labeling has

---

Journal of Sociology 61 (November 1955): 221–32. Moral crusaders are always obsessed with improving those whom they set out to benefit.

[29]Frank Tannenbaum, *Crime and the Community* (New York: Columbia Univ. Press, 1938).

[30]Wilbert Moore and Gerald W. Rosenblum, *The Professions: Roles and Rules* (New York: Russell Sage, 1970). See especially chap. 3 of this comprehensive guide to the literature, "The Professionalization of Occupations."

[31]William J. Goode, "Encroachment, Charlatanism, and the Emerging Professions: Psychology, Medicine, and Sociology," *American Sociological Review* 25 (December 1960): 902–14.

been medicalized to the point where all deviance has to have a medical label. The eclipse of the explicit moral component in medical diagnosis has thus invested Aesculapian authority[32] with totalitarian power.

The divorce between medicine and morality has been defended on the ground that medical categories, unlike those of law and religion, rest on scientific foundations exempt from moral evaluation.[33] Medical ethics have been secreted into a specialized department that brings theory into line with actual practice.[34] The courts and the law, when they are not used to enforce the Aesculapian monopoly, are turned into doormen of the hospital who select from among the clients those who can meet the doctors' criteria.[35] Hospitals turn into monuments of narcissistic scientism, concrete manifestations of those professional prejudices which were fashionable on the day their cornerstone was laid and which were often outdated when they came into use. The technical enterprise of the physician claims value-free power. It is obvious that in this kind of context it is easy to shun the issue of social iatrogenesis with which I am concerned. Politically medicated medical damage is thus seen as inherent in medicine's mandate, and its

---

[32]See Miriam Siegler and Humphrey Osmond, "Aesculapian Authority," *Hastings Center Studies* 1, no. 2 (1973): 41–52.

[33]Eliot Freidson, *Profession of Medicine: A Study of the Sociology of Applied Knowledge* (New York: Dodd, Mead, 1971), pp. 208 ff.

[34]June Goodfield, "Reflections on the Hippocratic Oaths," *Hastings Center Studies* 1, no. 2 (1973): 79–92.

[35]The law has had little experience with the problem of selecting one individual to live and thereby dooming others to die. Seamen have been convicted of manslaughter for having helped to throw 14 of 41 passengers out of a leaking lifeboat into the sea (*U.S.* vs. *Holmes,* 1842). So far the silence of the U.S. judiciary, combined with the silence of the legislature, seems to imply a preference for leaving decisions involving selection for survival to processes not subject to legal analysis. But increasing demands are made to create a rule of law to protect individuals seeking so-called life-prolonging treatment against the prejudices and arbitrariness of professional men. See below, note 204, p. 96.

critics are viewed as sophists trying to justify lay intrusion into the medical bailiwick. Precisely for this reason, a lay review of social iatrogenesis is urgent. The assertion of value-free cure and care is obviously malignant nonsense, and the taboos that have shielded irresponsible medicine are beginning to weaken.

The Medicalization of the Budget

The most handy measure of the medicalization of life is the share taken out of a typical yearly income to be spent under doctor's orders. In America before 1950, this was less than a month's income, but by the mid-seventies, the equivalent of between five and seven weeks of the typical worker's earnings were spent on the purchase of medical services. The United States now spends about $95 billion a year for health care, about 8.4 percent of the gross national product in 1975, up from 4.5 percent in 1962.[36] During the past twenty years, while the price index in the United States has risen by about 74 percent, the cost of medical care has escalated by 330 percent. Between 1950 and 1971 public expenditure for health insurance increased tenfold, private insurance benefits increased eightfold,[37] and direct out-of-pocket payments about

---

[36]Seymour E. Harris, *The Economics of American Medicine* (New York: Macmillan, 1964). A detailed survey of the cost of services, drugs, various levels of manpower, and hospitals; of historical value for the period between 1946 and 1961, during which health-care costs rose by 380%.

[37]Robert W. Hetherington, Carl E. Hopkins, and Milton I. Roemer, *Health Insurance Plans: Promise and Performance* (New York: Wiley 1975). The U.S. is dominated by a galaxy of autonomous and often competing health plans that are sometimes commercial, sometimes provider-sponsored, and sometimes organized along the lines of group practice. For most citizens all this is supplemented by some coverage through national health insurance. This evaluation of clients' reactions to different choices shows how little they really differ.

[38]Martin S. Feldstein, *The Rising Cost of Hospital Care* (Washington, D.C.: Information Resources, 1971). Hospital costs have outstripped by far the rise in physicians' fees. The over-all cost of medical care has gone up faster than the average cost of all goods

threefold.[38] In over-all expenditures other countries such as France[39] and Germany[40] kept abreast of the United States. In all industrial nations—Atlantic, Scandinavian, or East European—the growth rate of the health sector has advanced faster than that of the GNP.[41] Even discounting inflation, federal health outlays increased by more than 40 percent between 1969 and 1974.[42] The medicalization of the national budget, moreover, is not a privilege of the rich: in Colombia, a poor country that notoriously favors its rich, the proportion, as in England, is more than 10 percent.[43]

---

and services in the consumer price index. Prescription and drug costs have risen the least. Over-the-counter drug prices have actually fallen, but the drop is more than made up for by prescription costs.

[39]CREDOC (Centre de recherches et de documentation sur la consommation), *Évolution de la structure des soins médicaux, 1959–1972* (Paris, 1973).

[40]"Krankheitskosten: 'Die bombe tickt'; Das westdeutsche Gesundheitswesen," 1. "Der Kampf um die Kassen-Milliarden"; 2 "Die Phalanx der niedergelassenen Ärzte, " *Der Spiegel*, no. 19 (1975), pp. 54–66; no. 20 (1975), pp. 126–42.

[41]An excellent general introduction to the cost explosion in health care is R. Maxwell, *Health Care: The Proving Dilemma; Needs vs. Resources in Western Europe, the U.S., and the U.S.S.R.* (New York: McKinsey & Co., 1974). Ian Douglas-Wilson and Gordon McLachlan, eds., *Health Service Projects: An International Survey* (Boston: Little, Brown, 1973). This international comparison shows "the extreme heterogeneity in organization and ideology" of different systems. Everywhere "the rationalization is motivated, not by politics of the left or the right, but by the sheer necessity to secure more effective use of scarce and expensive resources." No country can indefinitely sustain unchecked increases in funds allocated for the treatment of illness.

[42]Louise Russell et al., *Federal Health Spending, 1969–74* (Washington, D.C.: Center for Health Policy Studies, National Planning Association, 1974). For comparison check B. Able Smith, *An International Study of Health Expenditures and Its Relevance for Health Planning,* Public Health Paper no. 32 (Geneva: World Health Organization, 1967). Based on a questionnaire to ministries, this supersedes the author's earlier *Paying for Health Services* and provides data for the study of trends. Herbert E. Klarman, *The Economics of Health* (New York: Columbia Univ. Press, 1965), gives a qualitative analysis of demand, supply, and organization in the U.S., with ample bibliographical guidance.

[43]John Bryant, *Health and the Developing World* (Ithaca, N.Y.: Cornell Univ. Press, 1969). A picture of health care in countries receiving international aid.

The phenomenal rise in cost of health services in the United States has been explained in different ways: some blame irrational planning,[51] others the higher cost of the new gimmicks that people want in hospitals.[52] The most common interpretation at present relates to the growing incidence of prepayment of services. Hospitals register well-insured patients, and rather than providing old products more efficiently and cheaply, are economically motivated to move towards new and increasingly expensive ways of doing things. Changing products rather than higher labor costs, bad administration, or lack of technological progress are blamed for the rise.[53] In this perspective the change in products seems due precisely to the increased insurance coverage which encourages hospitals to provide products more expensive than the customer actually wants, needs, or would have been willing to pay for directly. His out-of-pocket costs appear increasingly modest, even though the services offered by the hospital are more costly. Insurance for high-cost sick-care is thus a self-reinforcing process which invests the providers of care with the control of increasing resources.[54] As an antidote, some critics recommend enlightened cost con-

---

"average remaining lifetime" (ARL). It has remained nearly constant for 1947–1965, but the U.S. rate compared with other industrialized countries has fallen sharply for men and slightly for women. "There is no longer any significant relationship [in 30 countries studied] between the money spent on health and the longevity of the population." See also P. Longone, "Mortalité et morbidité," *Population et Société*, no. 43 (January 1972).

[51]Victor Cohen, "More Hospitals To Fill: Abuses Grow," *Technology Review*, October–November 1973, pp. 14–16.

[52]Robert F. Rushmer, *Medical Engineering: Projections for Health Care Delivery* (New York: Academic Press, 1972), expresses the hope that the forthcoming increase in federal funding will create a new market for spare parts, from breast-enhancers to artificial hearts.

[53]Feldstein, *Rising Cost of Hospital Care.*

[54]William A. Glaser, *Paying the Doctor: Systems of Remuneration and Their Effects* (Baltimore: Johns Hopkins, 1970). Consult this cross-national comparative analysis for the impact of different methods of payment on the costliness of the physician.

sciousness on the part of consumers;[55] others, not trusting the self-control of laymen, recommend mechanisms to heighten the cost consciousness of producers.[56] Physicians, they argue, would prescribe more responsibly and less wantonly if they were paid (as are general practitioners in Britain) on a "capitation" basis that provided a fixed amount for the maintenance of their clients rather than a fee for service. But like all other such remedies, capitation enlarges the iatrogenic fascination with the *health supply*. People forgo their own lives to get as much treatment as they can.

In England the National Health Service has tried, albeit unsuccessfully, to ensure that cost inflation will be less plagued by conspicuous flimflam.[57] The National Health Service Act of 1946 established access to health-care resources for all those in need as a human right. The need was assumed to be finite and quantifiable, the ballot box the best place to decide the total budget for health, and doctors the only ones able to determine the resources that would satisfy the need of each patient. But need as assessed by medical practitioners has proved to be just as extensive in England as anywhere else. The fundamental hope for the success of the English health-care system lay in the belief in the ability of the English to ration supply. Until about 1972 they did so, in the opinion of an author who surveyed British

---

[55]John and Sylvia Jewkes, *Value for Money in Medicine* (Oxford: Blackwell, 1963), pp. 30–7, argue: "It may be that, as electorates become more sophisticated, they will recognize they have in fact to pay for *free* services"; also that relatively cheap prevention through more healthy everyday habits is more effective than purchase of repairs.

[56]Fuchs, in *Who Shall Live?*, chap. 3, argues for institutional licensing as a substitute for the licensing of individuals. Under such a system, medical-care institutions would be licensed by the state and would then be free to hire and use personnel as each saw fit. This system would deploy resources more efficiently and provide more upward job mobility. But the physician's control over care produced and delivered by others would be weakened.

[57]For a bibliography on socialized medicine in Britain, consult Friedson, *Profession of Medicine*, p. 34, n. 9.

health economics, "by means in their way almost as ruthless—but generally held to be more acceptable—than the ability to pay."[58] Until that time health care was kept below 6 percent of GNP, 10 percent of public spending. Private practice had shrunk from half of all care to 4 percent. Direct charges to patients were kept at a phenomenally low 5 percent of the cost. But this stern commitment to equality prevented only those astounding misallocations for prestigious gadgetry which provided an easy starting point for public criticism in the United States. Since 1972 the Health Service in Britain has undergone a traumatic change, for complex economic and political reasons. The initial success of the Health Service and the present unique disarray in the system make predictions for the future impossible. Demedicalization of health care is as essential there as elsewhere. Yet curiously, England is also one of the few industrialized countries where the life expectancy of adult males has not yet declined, though the chronic diseases of this group have already shown an increase similar to that observed a decade earlier across the Atlantic.

Information on costs in the Soviet Union is more difficult to come by. The number of physicians and hospital days per capita seems to have doubled between 1960 and 1972, and costs to have increased by about 260 percent.[59] The main claim to superiority of Soviet medicine is still based on "prophylaxis built into the social system itself," without this affecting the relative volume of disease or care in comparison with other industrial countries of similar development.[60] But the theory that therapeutics would wither away

---

[58]Michael H. Cooper, *Rationing Health Care* (London: Halsted Press, 1975). A sober, critical, and lively attempt at an over-all economic review of the nature and problems of the first 26 years of the British National Health Service.

[59]Y. Lisitsin, *Health Protection in the USSR* (Moscow: Progress Publishers, 1972).

[60]Mark G. Field, *Soviet Socialized Medicine: An Introduction* (New York: Free Press, 1967). A standard introduction (now 12

with the state became and has remained heresy since 1932.[61]

Distinct political systems organize pathologies into different diseases and thus create distinct categories of demand, supply, and unmet needs.[62] But no matter how disease is perceived, the cost of treatment rises at comparable rates. The Russians, for instance, limit by decree mental disease requiring hospitalization: they allow only 10 percent of all hospital beds for such cases.[63] But at a given GNP all industrial nations generate the same kind of dependence on the physician, and do so irrespective of their ideology and the nosology these beliefs engender.[64] (Of course, capitalism has proved that it can do so at a much higher social cost.[65]) Everywhere in the mid-seventies the main constraint on professional activity is the necessity to reduce costs.

The proportion of national wealth which is channeled to doctors and expended under their control varies from one nation to another and falls somewhere between one-tenth and one-twentieth of all available funds. But this should lead nobody to believe that health expenditures on the typical citizen in poor countries are anywhere proportionate to the

---

years out of date) to the Soviet medical system. Pp. ix–xii provide a critical orientation to German, English, and French literature, and chap. 5, references to the return from social to curative priorities.

[61]See below, note 64.

[62]John Frey, *Medicine in Three Societies* (MTP, Aylesbury, England, 1974).

[63]Mark G. Field, "Soviet and American Approaches to Mental Illness: A Comparative Perspective," *Review of Soviet Medical Sciences* 1 (1964): 1–36.

[64]Joachim Israel, "Humanisierung oder Bürokratisierung der Medizin?" *Neue Gesellschaft* 21 (1974): 397–404. Provides an inventory of 15 strong tendencies towards the bureaucratization of life, which takes specifically health-related forms in medicine and menaces people equally in the Federal Republic of Germany and in the U.S.S.R.

[65]Odin W. Anderson, *Health Care: Can There Be Equity? The United States, Sweden, and England* (New York: Wiley, 1972). All three systems grow towards the same kind of bureaucracy, at comparable costs, but equity in access is much lower in the U.S.A.

countries' per capita average income. Most people get absolutely nothing. Excepting only the money allocated for treatment of water supplies, 90 percent of all funds earmarked for health in developing countries is spent not for sanitation but for treatment of the sick. From 70 percent to 80 percent of the entire *public* health budget goes to the cure and care of individuals as opposed to public health services.[66] Most of this money is spent *everywhere* on the same kinds of things.

All countries want hospitals, and many want them to have the most exotic modern equipment. The poorer the country, the higher the real cost of each item on their inventories. Modern hospital beds, incubators, laboratories, respirators, and operating rooms cost even more in Africa than their counterparts in Germany or France where they are manufactured: they also break down more easily in the tropics, are more difficult to service, and are more often than not out of use. As to cost, the same is true of the physicians who are made to measure for these gadgets. The education of an open-heart surgeon represents a comparable capital investment, whether he comes from the Mexican school system or is the cousin of a Brazilian captain sent on a government scholarship to study in Hamburg.[67] The United States might be

---

[66]International Bank for Reconstruction and Development, *Health Sector Policy Paper*, Washington, D.C., March 1975.

[67]It must not be overlooked that medical schools in poor countries constitute one of the most effective means for the net transfer of money to the rich countries. O. Ozlak and D. Caputo, "The Migration of Medical Personnel from Latin America to the U.S.: Towards an Alternative Interpretation," paper presented at the Pan-American Conference on Health and Manpower Planning, Ottawa, Canada, September 10–14, 1973. The authors estimate that the *annual* net loss for the whole of Latin America due to the flow of physicians to the U.S. is $200 million, a figure equal to the total medical aid given by the U.S. to Latin America during the first development decade, i.e., the period that started with the "Alliance for Progress." Hossain A. Ronaghy, Kathleen Cahill, and Timothy D. Baker, "Physician Migration to the United States: One Country's Transfusion Is Another Country's Hemorrhage," *Journal of the American Medical Association* 227 (1974): 538–42, provides infor-

too poor to provide renal dialysis at $15,000 per year to all those citizens who would claim to need it, but Ghana is too poor to provide the people equitably with physicians for primary care.[68] Socially critical maximum cost of items that can be equitably shared varies from one place to another. But whenever tax funds are used to finance treatment above the critical cost, the system of medical care acts inevitably as a device for the net transfer of power from the majority who pay the taxes to the few who are selected because of their money, schooling, or family ties, or because of their special interest to the experimenting surgeon.

It is clearly a form of exploitation when four-fifths of the real cost of *private* clinics in poor Latin American countries is paid for by the taxes collected for medical education, public ambulances, and medical equipment.[69] In this case the concentration of public resources on a few is obviously unjust because

---

mation on outmigration of Iranian students by the university from which they graduated. Oscar Gish, ed., *Doctor Migration and World Health,* Occasional Papers on Social Administration no. 43, Social Administration Research Trust (London: Bell, 1971). Stephen S. Mick, "The Foreign Medical Graduate," *Scientific American* 232 (February 1975): 14–22. There are 58,000 imported physicians now practicing in the U.S.; fully licensed practitioners have quadrupled. In the Middle Atlantic, North Central, and New England regions, they outnumber native physicians. India, the Philippines, Italy, and Canada each paid for the full education of more than 3,000 of these; Argentina, South Korea, and Thailand, among others, for more than 1,000 each. N.B.: The training of a Peruvian physician costs about six thousand times as much as the education of a typical Peruvian peasant.

[68]In Ghana, the Central Hospital absorbed 149 of the 298 physicians available to the official health services, yet only about 1% of the patients had been officially referred by medical personnel outside the hospital. M. J. Sharpston, "Uneven Geographical Distribution of Medical Care, a Ghanaian Case Study," *Journal of Development Studies* 8 (January 1972): 205–22.

[69]For a useful survey of social research on health in Latin America, see Arthur Rubel, "The Role of Social Science Research in Recent Health Programs in Latin America," *Latin American Research Review* 2 (1966): 37–56. Dieber Zschock, "Health Planning in Latin America: Review and Evaluation," *Latin American Research Review* 5 (1970): 35–56.

the ability to pay out of pocket a fraction of the total cost of treatment is a condition for getting the rest underwritten. But the exploitation is no less in places where the public, through a national health service, assigns to physicians the sole power to decide who "needs" their kind of treatment, and then lavishes public support on those on whom they experiment or practice. The public acquiescence in the doctor's monopoly on identifying needs only broadens the base from which doctors can sell their services.[70]

Indirectly, conspicuous therapies serve as powerful devices to convince people that they should pay more taxes to get them to all those whom doctors have declared in need. Once President Frei of Chile had started on one palace for medical spectator-sports, his successor, Salvador Allende, was forced to promise three more. The prestige of a puny national team in the medical Olympics is used to intensify a nationwide addiction to therapeutic relationships that are pathogenic on a level much deeper than mere medical vandalism. More health damage is caused by people's belief that they cannot cope with their illness unless they call on the doctor than doctors could ever cause by foisting their ministrations on people.

Only in China—at least, at first sight—does the trend seem to run in the opposite direction: primary care is given by nonprofessional health technicians assisted by health apprentices who leave their regular jobs in the factory when they are called on to assist a member of their brigade.[71] Nutrition, environmental

---

[70]Victor R. Fuchs, "The Contribution of Health Services to the American Economy," *Milbank Memorial Fund Quarterly* 44 (October 1966): 65–103. Fuchs drives this point home.

[71]For orientation see Joshua Horn, *Away with All Pests: An English Surgeon in People's China, 1954–1969* (New York: Monthly Review Press, 1971). Victor W. and Ruth Sidel, "Medicine in China: Individual and Society," *Hastings Center Studies* 2, no. 3 (1974): 23–36. Victor Sidel, "The Barefoot Doctors of the People's Republic of China," *New England Journal of Medicine* 286 (1972): 1292–1300. A. J. Smith, "Medicine in China" (5 articles), *British Medical Journal,* 1974, 2:367–70, and the following four issues. Carl Djerassi, "The Chinese Achievement in Fertility Con-

hygiene, and birth control have improved beyond comparison. The achievements in the Chinese health sector during the late sixties have proved, perhaps definitively, a long-debated point: that almost all demonstrably effective technical health devices can be taken over within months and used competently by millions of ordinary people. Despite such successes, an orthodox commitment to Western dreams of reason in Marxist shape may now destroy what political virtue combined with traditional pragmatism, has achieved. The bias towards technological progress and centralization is reflected already in the professional reaches of medical care. China possesses not only a paramedical system but also medical personnel whose educational standards are known to be of the highest order by their counterparts around the world, and which differ only marginally from those of other countries. Most investment during the last four years seems to have gone towards the further development of this extremely well qualified and highly orthodox medical profession, which is getting increasing authority to shape the over-all health goals of the nation. "Barefoot medicine" is losing its makeshift, semi-independent, grassroots character and is being integrated into a unitary health-care technocracy. University-trained personnel instruct, supervise, and complement the locally elected healer. This ideologically fueled development of professional medicine in China will have to be consciously limited in the very near future if it is to remain a balancing complement rather than an

---

trol," *Bulletin of the Atomic Scientists*, June 1974, pp. 17–24. Paul T. K. Lin, "Medicine in China," *Center Magazine* (Santa Barbara, Calif.), May–June, 1974. M. H. Liang et al., "Chinese Health Care: Determinants of the System," *American Journal of Public Health* 63 (February 1973): 102–10. Horn's is still the best first-person report. Sidel's and Smith's are reports from traveling colleagues to the profession. Djerassi gives valuable insights into the status of contraception. Lin calls attention to the new challenges created by the recent prevalence of degenerative disease. See also Ralph C. Croizier, *Traditional Medicine in Modern China: Science, Nationalism, and the Tension of Cultural Change* (Cambridge: Harvard Univ. Press, 1968).

obstacle to high-level self-care.[72] Without comparable statistics, statements on Chinese medical economy remain vague. But there is no reason to believe that cost increases in pharmaceutical, hospital, and professional medicine in China are less than in other countries. For the time being, however, it can be argued that in China modern medicine in rural districts was so scarce that recent increments contributed significantly to health levels and to increased equity in access to care.[73]

In all countries the medicalization of the budget is related to well-recognized exploitation within the class structure. No doubt, the dominance of capitalist oligarchies in the United States,[74] the superciliousness of the new mandarins in Sweden,[75] the ser-

---

[72]David Lampton, *Health, Conflict, and the Chinese Political System,* Michigan Papers in Chinese Studies no. 18 (Ann Arbor: Univ. of Michigan, Center for Chinese Studies, 1974). Since 1971 competing interest groups, each trying to maximize realization of its values, have helped to re-establish the pre-1968 bureaucratic model in medicine.

[73]Instruments for the further study of contemporary Chinese health care: Joseph Quinn, *Medicine and Public Health in the People's Republic of China,* U.S. Department of Health, Education, and Welfare no. NIH 73–67. Fogarty International Center, *A Bibliography of Chinese Sources on Medicine and Public Health in the People's Republic of China: 1960–1970,* Department of Health, Education, and Welfare publication no. NIH 73–439. *American Journal of Chinese Medicine,* P.O. Box 555, Garden City, N.Y. 11530.

[74]Vicente Navarro, "The Underdevelopment of Health or the Health of Underdevelopment: An Analysis of the Distribution of Human Health Resources in Latin America," *International Journal of Health Services* 4, no. 1 (1974): 5–27. Scarcity of health care is consistent with the general scarcity of industrial output that favors an urban, entrepreneurial *lumpen*-bourgeoisie dependent on its foreign counterparts. This paper is based on a presentation at the Pan-American Conference on Health and Manpower Planning in Ottawa, Canada, September 10–14, 1973. A modified version appears in the spring 1974 issue of *Politics and Society.*

[75]B. Shenkin, "Politics and Medical Care in Sweden: The Seven Crowns Reform," *New England Journal of Medicine* 288 (1973): 555–59. For background consult Ronald Huntford, *The New Totalitarians* (New York: Stein & Day, 1972).

vility and ethnocentrism of Moscow professionals,[76] and the lobby of the American Medical and Pharmaceutical Associations,[77] as well as the new rise of union power in the health sector,[78] are all formidable obstacles to a distribution of resources in the interests of the sick rather than of their self-appointed caretakers. But the fundamental reason why these costly bureaucracies are health-denying lies not in their instrumental but in their symbolic function: they all stress delivery of repair and maintenance services for the human component of the megamachine,[79] and criticism that proposes better and more equitable delivery only reinforces the social commitment to keep people at work in sickening jobs. The war between the proponents of unlimited national health insurance and those who stand up for national health maintenance, as well as the war between those defending and those attacking all private practice, shifts public attention from the damage done by doctors who protect a destructive social order to the fact that doctors

---

[76]Roy A. and Zhores Medvedev, *A Question of Madness* (New York: Knopf, 1972), complain that the nature of society is such that at least two professions, medicine and law, are not part of the state system. The totalitarian centralization of medical services, while it has introduced the progressive principle of free health care for all, has also made it possible to use medicine as a means of government control and political regulation.

[77]David R. Hyde et al., "The American Medical Association: Power, Purpose, and Politics in Organized Medicine," *Yale Law Journal* 63 (May 1954): 938–1022. Hyde is an early, dated, but still valuable critic. Richard Harris, *A Sacred Trust* (Baltimore: Penguin, 1969). A history of the American Medical Association's clever and costly battle against public health legislation in the sixties. Elton Rayack, *Professional Power and American Medicine: The Economics of the American Medical Association* (Cleveland: World Pub., 1967), describes blackmail and conspiracy by the American Medical Association lobby to maintain tight control over licensing and the setting of standards for every product that physicians perceive as health-related. This control removes all limits from their power.

[78]On the reasons that foreshadow the unionization of doctors, see S. Kelman, "Towards a Political Economy of Medical Care," *Inquiry* 8, no. 3 (1971): 30–8; also note 79, p. 245.

[79]Lewis Mumford, *The Pentagon of Power*, vol. 2, *The Myth of the Machine* (New York: Harcourt Brace, 1970), elaborates on the concept of society as megamachine.

do less than expected in defense of a consumer society.

Beyond a certain encroachment on the budget, money that expands medical control over space, schedules, education, diet, or the design of machines and goods will inevitably unleash a "nightmare forged from good intentions." Money may always threaten health. Too much money corrupts it. Beyond a certain point, what can produce money or what money can buy restricts the range of self-chosen "life." Not only production but also consumption stresses the scarcity of time, space, and choice.[80] Therefore the prestige of medical staples must sap the cultivation of health, which, within a given environment, to a large extent depends on innate and inbred mettle.[81] The more time, toil, and sacrifice spent by a population in producing medicine as a commodity, the larger will be the by-product, namely, the fallacy that society has a supply of *health* locked away which can be mined and marketed.[82] The negative function

---

[80]Beyond a certain point of intensity, consumption produces a scarcity of time: Staffan B. Linder, *Harried Leisure Class* (New York: Columbia Univ. Press, 1970); acceleration produces a penury of space: Jean Robert, "Essai sur l'accélération des dons," *L'Arc* (Aix-en-Provence), fall 1975; and planning destroys the possibilities for choice: Herbert Marcuse, *Eros and Civilization* (Boston: Beacon Press, 1955).

[81]René Dubos, *Man and His Environment: Biomedical Knowledge and Social Action,* Pan-American Health Organization, Scientific Publication no. 131 (Washington, D.C., March 1966). "The kind of health that men desire most is . . . the condition best suited to reach goals that each individual formulates for himself." See also Heinz von Foerster, *Molecular Ethology: An Immodest Proposal* (New York: Plenum Press, 1970), for a demonstration from theoretical biology that nontrivial "life" can be extinguished by overprogramming.

[82]Victor Fuchs, "Some Economic Aspects of Mortality in Developed Countries," paper presented at the Conference on the Economy of Health and Medical Care, Tokyo, 1973, mimeographed. Fuchs assumes that "life is primarily produced by nonmarket activities, and that the female tends to specialize in such activities." The attempt to replace rather than to complement these "nonmarket activities" with commodities is literally *unhealthy.* See Alan Berg, *The Nutrition Factor: Its Role in National Development* (Washington, D.C.: Brookings Institution, 1973), app. C, p. 229, on the sickening effects of the substitution of various formulas for breast milk.

of money is that of an indicator of the devaluation of goods and services that cannot be bought.[83] The higher the price tag at which well-being is commandeered, the greater will be the political prestige of an expropriation of personal health.

The Pharmaceutical Invasion

Doctors are not needed to *medicalize* a society's drugs.[84] Even without too many hospitals and medical schools a culture can become the prey of a pharmaceutical invasion. Each culture has its poisons, its remedies, its placebos, and its ritual settings for their administration.[85] Most of these are destined for the

---

[83]The medicalization of the budget is a measure of the professional *disseizin* of health and of the acquiescence of people in their own disendowment by therapeutic caretakers. *Disseizin:* "the wrongful putting out of him from that which is actually seized as a freehold": P. G. Osborn, *Concise Law Dictionary* (London: Sweet & Maxwell, 1964).

[83a]Jean Pierre Dupuy, Serge Karsenty. L'invasion pharmaceutique. Paris, Seuil 1974 . . . have created this term. They describe the mutual re-inforcement of three forces: unrealistic expectations on the part of patient-majorities; the medical management of a technical system having primarily symbolic functions; and the advertising of pseudo-inventions that constitutes an ever larger share of activities performed by the pharmaceutical industry. The three forces converge as a back-up for capital-accumulation in the health sector.

The author is profoundly indebted to Dupuy and Karsenty for their collaboration on the French draft of this book.

[84]For a first orientation: Alfred M. Ajami, Jr., *Drugs: An Annotated Bibliography and Guide to the Literature* (Boston: Hall, 1973). Ajami selects and annotates more than 500 references on psychopharmacology for an interdisciplinary course on the U.S. "scene" of the late sixties. U.S. National Clearing House for Mental Health, *Bibliography of Drug Dependence and Abuse 1928–1966* (Chevy Chase, Md., 1969). Indispensable for historical research. Alice L. Brunn, *How to Find Out in Pharmacy: A Guide to Sources of Pharmaceutical Information* (Oxford: Pergamon Press, 1969). A simple reference guide. R. H. Blum et al., *Society and Drugs,* 2 vols. (Berkeley, Calif.: Jossey-Bass, 1970). A portable library on society and drugs.

[85]G. E. Vaillant, "The Natural History of Narcotic Drug Addiction," in *Seminars in Psychiatry* 2 (November 1970): 486–98. Drugs depend both for their desirability and their effect on the milieu in which they are taken. The choice of the drug is a function

healthy rather than for the sick.[86] Powerful medical drugs easily destroy the historically rooted pattern that fits each culture to its poisons; they usually cause more damage than profit to health, and ultimately establish a new attitude in which the body is perceived as a machine run by mechanical and manipulating switches.[87]

In the 1940s few of the prescriptions written in Houston or Madrid could have been filled in Mexico, except in the *zona rosa* of Mexico City, where international pharmacies flourish alongside boutiques and hotels. Today Mexican village drugstores offer three times as many items as drugstores in the United States.

---

of the culture, but the abuse of the drug is a function of the man. The ritualization of drug-taking creates its subculture: thus the history of drug addiction as that of society must be rewritten every few years. Samuel Proger, ed., *The Medicated Society* (New York: MacMillan, 1968), provides documents showing the kind of drug culture that prevailed in the U.S. long before LSD.

The extent to which addicts are forced into a ghetto of their own depends upon the community that rejects them. For instance, Puerto Ricans in New York do not reject their addicts in the way middle-class Americans do: J. P. Fitzpatrick, "Puerto Rican Addicts and Nonaddicts: A Comparison," unpublished report, Institute for Social Research, Fordham University, 1975.

[86]Hans Wiswe, *Kulturgeschichte der Kochkunst: Kochbücher und Rezepte aus zwei Jahrtausenden* (Munich: Moos, 1970). Most societies cannot distinguish clearly between their pharmacopeia and their diet. This survey of cookbooks shows that many were written by physicians, with a frequent insistence that the best medicine comes from the kitchen and not from the pharmacy. Most contain "recipes" for the care of the sick.

[87]For the present information available on drug action, see Louis S. Goodman and Alfred Gilman, *The Pharmacological Basis of Therapeutics*, 4th ed. (New York: Macmillan, 1970). On prescribing patterns, see Karen Dunnell and Ann Cartwright, *Medicine Takers, Prescribers and Hoarders* (London: Routledge, 1972). Who takes which sort of medicines for what types of conditions and symptoms? How do doctors encourage or discourage this pattern? What kinds of medicines are kept in the home and for how long? Detailed information about England. Also see John P. Morgan and Michael Weintraub, "A Course on the Social Functions of Prescription Drugs: Seminar Syllabus and Bibliography," *Annals of Internal Medicine* 77 (August 1972): 217–22; Paul Stolley and Louis Lasagna, "Prescribing Patterns of Physicians," *Journal of Chronic Diseases* 22 (December 1969): 395–405.

In Thailand[88] and Brazil, many items that are elsewhere outdated, or illegal surplus and duds, are dumped into pharmacies by manufacturers who sail under many flags of convenience. In the past decade, while a few rich countries began to control the damage, waste, and exploitation caused by the *licit* drug-pushing of their doctors, physicians in Mexico, Venezuela, and even Paris had more difficulty than ever before in getting information on the side-effects of the drugs they prescribed.[89] Only ten years ago, when drugs were relatively scarce in Mexico, people were poor, and most sick persons were attended by grandmother or the herbalist, pharmaceuticals came packaged with a descriptive leaflet. Today drugs are more plentiful, more powerful, and more dangerous; they are sold by television and radio; people who have attended school feel ashamed of their lingering trust in the Aztec curer; and the leaflet has been replaced by one standard note which says, "on prescription." The fiction which is meant to exorcise the drug by medicalizing it in fact only confounds the buyer. The warning to consult a doctor makes the buyer believe he is incompetent to beware. In most countries of the world, doctors are simply not well enough spread out to prescribe double-edged medicine each time it is indicated, and most of the time they themselves are not prepared, or are too ignorant, to prescribe with due prudence. As a consequence the physician's function, especially in poor countries, has become trivial: he has been turned into a routine prescription machine that is constantly ridiculed, and

---

[88]*Business in Thailand*, special issue on the pharmaceutical industry, August 1974.

[89]The American physician can easily gain access to this information from such sources as *Medical Letter on Drugs and Therapeutics*, Medical Library Association, 919 N. Michigan Avenue, Chicago, Ill. This is an unbiased source of drug information mailed fortnightly. Nothing comparable is available in French, German, or Spanish. Also see Richard Burack, *The New Handbook of Prescription Drugs: Official Names, Prices, and Sources for Patient and Doctor*, rev. ed. (New York: Pantheon, 1970.) (See below, note 99, p. 61, for description of this book.)

most people now take the same drugs, just as haphazardly, but without his approval.[90]

Chloramphenicol is a good example of the way reliance on prescription can be useless for the protection of patients and can even promote abuse. During the 1960s this drug was packaged as Chloromycetin by Parke, Davis and brought in about one-third of the company's over-all profits. By then it had been known for several years that people who take this drug stand a certain chance of dying of aplastic anemia, an incurable disease of the blood. Typhoid is almost the only disease that, with serious qualifications, does justify the taking of this substance. Through the late fifties and early sixties, Parke, Davis, notwithstanding strong clinical contraindications, spent large sums to promote their winner. Doctors in the United States prescribed chloramphenicol to almost four million people per year to treat them for acne, sore throat, the common cold, and even such trifles as infected hangnail. Since typhoid is rare in the United States, no more than one in 400 of those given the drug "needed" the treatment. Unlike thalidomide, which disfigures, chloramphenicol kills: it puts its victims out of sight, and hundreds of them in the United States died undiagnosed.[91]

---

[90]In most cultures people remained dependent on remedies collected by a member of the family in the woods or grown on the window-sill. This even occurred in societies where subsistence-production had ceded to the market in many other areas. Throughout millennia, the world trade in drugs was conducted by peddlers and had "nothing in common with bourgeois, commercial trade, however much many historical philologists may wish to establish the reverse." On this see J. C. van Leur, Indonesian Trade and Society: Essays in Asian Social and Economic History. (The Hague; van Hoeve Publ., 1967) esp. 45–88. On the trade in medical, technical, cosmetic and religious chemicals in antiquity see: Alfred Schmidt. Drogen und Drogen-handel im Altertum. (Leipzig. J.A. Barth, 1924) Wolfgang-Hagen Hein, Christus als Apotheker. (Frankfurt; Govi Verlag, 1947) shows how Christ in German paintings turned quite suddenly around 1700 from the celestial healer of human disease into the heavenly apothecary dispensing spiritual merchandise.

[91]The information on Chloromycetin is taken from U.S. Senate, Select Committee on Small Business, Subcommittee on Monopoly,

Self-control by the profession on such matters has never worked,[92] and medical memories have proved particularly short.[93] The best one can say is that in Holland or Norway or Denmark, self-regulation has at certain moments been less ineffective than in Germany or France[94] or Italy,[95] and that American doctors have a particular facility for admitting past mistakes and jumping on new bandwagons.[96] In the United States in the fifties, control over drugs by regulatory agencies was at a low ebb and self-control was nominal.[97] Then, during the sixties, concerned newspapermen,[98] medical men,[99] and politicians[100] launched a

---

Competitive Problems in the Drug Industry, 90th Congress, 1st and 2nd Sessions, 1967–68, pt. 2, p. 565.

[92]On the mechanisms that turn self-regulation into license for performance of the maximum publically tolerated abuse, see Eliot Friedson and Buford Rhea, "Process of Control in a Company of Equals," *Social Problems* 9 (1963): 119–131. They show that, though much abuse goes unobserved, even if observed it is not communicated to colleagues, and even if communicated it is treated by "talking to the offender" and remains uncontrolled. Self-regulation principally protects the profession by eliminating the incompetent butcher and the brazen moral leper. William J. Goode, "The Protection of the Inept," *American Sociological Review* 32 (February 1967): 5–19. Goode describes how self-regulation consists to a large degree in the protection of the inept within the group and the protection of the group's self-interest from the excesses of the inept. Modernization consists in the more efficient utilization of the inept in the self-interest of the group. Eliot Freidson and Buford Rhea, "Knowledge and Judgment in Professional Evaluations," *Administrative Science Quarterly* 10 (June 1965): 107–24.

[93]Memory is no guide to which drugs have been prescribed or consumed in the past. A search in the national registry of prescriptions in England and Wales show that 8 out of 10 women who had borne a defective child after taking thalidomide on prescription denied that they had taken the drug, and that their physicians denied having ordered it. See A. L. Speirs, "Thalidomide and Congenital Abnormalities," *Lancet,* 1962, 1:303.

[94]Henri Pradal, *Guide des médicaments les plus courants* (Paris: Seuil, 1974). In November 1973 my French publisher, Seuil, brought out a paperback original of this book by a physician with many years' experience as a toxicologist. It is a list of the 100 best-selling pharmaceuticals, including prescription drugs, explaining what each one is, what it is indicated for, how it tends to be used or prescribed, and with what consequences. On publication day 57 drug firms started separate legal actions to have the book withdrawn and sued for reimbursement for probable damages.

[95]A. del Favero and G. Loiacono, *Farmaci, salute e profitti in Italia* (Milan: Feltrinelli, 1974), describe the dependence and ser-

campaign that exposed the subservience of physicians and government officials to pharmaceutical firms and described some of the prevalent patterns of white-collar crimes in medicine.[101] Within two months after

---

vility of the Italian physician in his relations with the drug industry, and the exploitative integration of the Italian drug firms among transnational companies. Full of documentation and detail.

[96]James H. Young, *Medical Messiahs: A Social History of Health Quackery in Twentieth-Century America* (Princeton, N.J.: Princeton Univ. Press, 1967). Historical background for the cavalier confidence of U.S. organized medicine based on its protection of the public against free-lance healers and self-medication. For the earlier history see James H. Young, *The Toadstool Millionaires: A Social History of Patent Medicines in America Before Federal Regulation* (Princeton, N.J.: Princeton Univ. Press, 1961).

[97]Robert S. McCleery, *One Life—One Physician: An Inquiry into the Medical Profession's Performance in Self-Regulation*, A Report to the Center for the Study of Responsive Law (Washington, D.C.: Public Affairs Press, 1971). This report to a study group initiated by Ralph Nader concludes that there is a total lack of internal quality control within the medical profession.

[98]Morton Mintz, *By Prescription Only: A Report on the Roles of the United States Food and Drug Administration, the American Medical Association, Pharmaceutical Manufacturers and Others in Connection with the Irrational and Massive Use of Prescription Drugs That May Be Worthless, Injurious, or Even Lethal*, 2nd ed. (Boston: Beacon Press, 1967). Originally published as *The Therapeutic Nightmare* (Boston: Houghton Mifflin, 1965), this masterpiece of investigative journalism by a staff reporter of the *Washington Post* has done more than any other book to change the focus of the U.S. discussion of medicine. For ten years a benevolent minority had worried about the damage done by capitalist medicine to the poor. Now the pill-swallowing majority became aware of what it was doing to them.

[99]Richard Burack, M.D., *The New Handbook of Prescription Drugs: Official Names, Prices and Sources for Patient and Doctor* (New York: Pantheon, 1970). Published at a time when judicial evidence for the undue bias of regulatory commissions, conspiracy for the dissemination of misleading information on poisonous drugs, and the venality of not a few professors of medicine was still difficult to obtain this book provides information and evaluation of the efficiency, usefulness, side-effects, and application of the 200 most prescribed drugs, comments on brand-name prices in comparison with generic equivalents (for which suppliers are listed with addresses), and adds spicy anecdotes on many trademarked nostrums.

[100]James L. Goddard, "The Drug Establishment," *Esquire*, March 1969. A readable and well-researched report.

[101]Edwin Sutherland, *White-Collar Crime* (New York: Holt, 1961), uses this term to designate a wide variety of serious offenses involving recognized social harm that either are not prosecuted or are confined to civil courts. The medical variety has epidemic consequences and might be called "white-coat crime."

the exposure at a congressional hearing, the use of chloramphenicol in the United States dwindled. Parke-Davis was forced to insert strict warnings of hazards and cautionary statements about the use of this drug into every package. But these warnings did not extend to exports.[102] The drug continued to be used indiscriminately in Mexico, not only in self-medication but on prescription, thereby breeding a drug-resistant strain of typhoid bacilli which is now spreading from Central America to the rest of the world.

One doctor in Latin America who was also a statesman did try to stem the pharmaceutical invasion rather than just enlist physicians to make it look more respectable. During his short tenure as president of Chile, Dr. Salvador Allende[103] quite successfully mobilized the poor to identify their own health needs and much less successfully compelled the medical profession to serve basic rather than profitable needs. He proposed to ban drugs unless they had been tried on paying clients in North America or Europe for as long as the patent protection would run. He revived a program aimed at reducing the national pharmacopeia to a few dozen items, more or less the same as those carried by the Chinese barefoot doctor in his black wicker box. Notably, within one week after the Chilean military junta took power on September 11,

---

[102]Herbert Schreier and Lawrence Berger, "On Medical Imperialism: A Letter," *Lancet*, 1974, 1:1161: "Under pressure from the US Food and Drug Administration, Parke-Davis inserted strict warnings of hazards and cautionary statements about indications for the use of the drug in the USA. The warning did not extend to the same drug abroad." Also see John F. Hellergers, "Chloramphenicol in Japan: Let It Bleed," *Bulletin of Concerned Asia Scholars* 5 (July 1973): 37–45. The expansion of federal controls over the export of *drugs* would only partially remedy this form of imperialism. Federal authority, which now does cover the $6 billion pharmaceutical drug industry, does not yet extend over the $3 billion *medical device* industry. It cannot, for example, stop the A. H. Robins company from supplying foreign companies with a model of a contraceptive shield which has been withdrawn from the U.S. market because of its high infection rate; see *Hastings Center Studies* 5, no. 3 (1975): 2.

[103]On medicine in Chile under Allende consult Howard Waitzkin and Hilary Modell, "Medicine, Socialism, and Totalitarianism:

1973, many of the most outspoken proponents of a Chilean medicine based on community rather than on drug imports and drug consumption had been murdered.[104]

The overconsumption of medical drugs is, of course, not restricted to areas where doctors are scarce or people are poor. In the United States, the volume of the drug business has grown by a factor of 100 during the current century:[105] 20,000 tons of aspirin are consumed per year, almost 225 tablets per person.[106] In England, every tenth night of sleep is induced by a hypnotic drug and 19 percent of women and 9 percent of men take a prescribed tranquilizer during any one year.[107] In the United States, central-nervous-system agents are the fastest-growing sector of the pharmaceutical market, now making up 31

Lesson from Chile," *New England Journal of Medicine* 291 (1974): 171–7; Vicente Navarro, "What Does Chile Mean? An Analysis of Events in the Health Sector Before, During, and After Allende's Administration," *Milbank Memorial Fund Quarterly* 52 (spring 1974): 93–130. This article is based on a paper presented at the International Health Seminar at Harvard University, February 1974. For an eyewitness report, see Ursula Bernauer and Elisabeth Freitag, *Poder popular in Chile am Beispiel Gesundheit: Dokumente aus Elendsvierteln* (Stein/Nuremberg: Laetere/Imba, 1974).

[104]Albert Jonsen et al., "Doctors in Politics: A Lesson from Chile," *New England Journal of Medicine* 291 (1974): 471–2. Describes the particular violence with which physicians were persecuted by the junta.

[105]John M. Firestone, *Trends in Prescription Drug Prices* (Washington, D.C.: Enterprise Institute for Public Policy Research, 1970). Drug expenditures account for only about 10% of health expenditures. The moderate rise in the cost of each prescription during the last years is due mainly to an increase in the size of the average prescription.

[106]Edward M. Brecher and Consumer Reports Editors, *Licit and Illicit Drugs: The Consumers Union Report on Narcotics, Stimulants, Depressants, Inhalants, Hallucinogens and Marijuana—Including Caffeine, Nicotine and Alcohol* (Boston: Little, Brown, 1973).

[107]D. M. Dunlop, "The Use and Abuse of Psychotropic Drugs," in *Proceedings of the Royal Society of Medicine* 63 (1970): 1279. G. L. Klerman, "Social Values and the Consumption of Psychotropic Medicine," in *Proceedings of the First World Congress on Environmental Medicine and Biology* (Haarlem: North-Holland, 1974). For a particularly pernicious form of medically prescribed drug addiction see Dorothy Nelkin, *Methadone Maintenance: A Technological Fix* (New York: Braziller, 1973).

percent of total sales.[108] Dependence on prescribed tranquilizers has risen by 290 percent since 1962, a period during which the per capita consumption of liquor rose by only 23 percent and the estimated consumption of illegal opiates by about 50 percent.[109] A significant quantity of "uppers" and "downers" is obtained in all countries by circumventing the doctor.[110] Medicalized addiction[111] in 1975 has out-grown all self-chosen or more festive forms of creating well-being.[112]

---

[108]James L. Goddard, "The Medical Business," *Scientific American* 229 (September 1973): 161–6. Contains graphs and charts showing U.S. sales of prescription and nonprescription drugs by category, 1962–71; breakdown by sales dollar estimated in 1968 for 17 leading pharmaceutical houses; introduction of new drugs, combinations, and dosage forms, 1958–72. Also identifies 8 classes of prescription drugs. Within the category "nervous system drugs" alone, sales aggregate more than $1 billion per year. This compares with three other categories each aggregating about $500 million, and the rest, each less than $350 million. For a breakdown, by age, sex, and type, of medicines prescribed to nonhospitalized patients in the course of one year in the U.S., see B. S. H. Harris and J. B. Hallan, "The Number and Cost of Prescribed Medicines: Selected Diseases," *Inquiry* 7 (1970): 38–50.

[109]*Drug Use in America: Problem in Perspective,* Second Report of the National Commission on Marihuana and Drug Abuse, 1972, 1973, 1974, 4 vols. (Washington, D.C.: Government Printing Office; stock no. 5266-0003). National Commission for the Study of Nursing and Nursing Education, *An Abstract for Action* (New York: McGraw-Hill, 1970).

[110]Mitchell Balter et al., "Cross-national Study of the Extent of Anti-Anxiety/Sedative Drug Use," *New England Journal of Medicine* 290 (1974): 769–74.

[111]Michael Balint, *Treatment or Diagnosis: A Study of Repeat Prescriptions in General Practice,* Mind and Medicine Monographs (Philadelphia: Lippincott, 1970). Prescription provides luster and seeming rationality to the belief that progress consists in buying one's way out of everything, including reality itself. Balint points out that in two-thirds of cases in which drugs were repeatedly prescribed without any technical justification, the physician himself took the initiative to offer the drug. Harry Dowling, "How Do Practicing Physicians Use New Drugs?" *Journal of the American Medical Association* 185 (1963): 233–36. Out of fear of "doing nothing" the practitioner is led to prescribe more than is indicated by instructions on the package. On the pattern according to which prescription abuses spread, see Leighton E. Cluff et al., "Studies in the Epidemiology of Adverse Drug Reactions," *Journal of the American Medical Association* 188 (1964): 976–83.

[112]Philippe de Félice, *Poisons sacrés: Ivresses divines; Essai sur quelques formes inférieures de la mystique* (Paris: Albin, 1936; re-

It has become fashionable to blame multinational pharmaceutical firms for the increase in medically prescribed drug abuse; their profits are high and their control over the market is unique. For fifteen years, drug industry profits (as a percentage of sales and company net worth) have outranked those of all other manufacturing industries listed on the Stock Exchange. Drug prices are controlled and manipulated: the same bottle that sells for two dollars in Chicago or Geneva where it is produced, but where it faces competition, sells for twelve dollars in a poor country where it does not.[113] The markup, moreover, is phenomenal: forty dollars' worth of diazepam, once stamped into pills and packaged as Valium, sells for a range of high prices, some as much as 70 times that of phenobarbital, which, in the opinion of most pharmacologists, has the same indications, effects, and dangers.[114] As commodities, prescription drugs behave differently from most other items: they are products that the ultimate consumer rarely selects for himself.[115] The producer's sales efforts are directed at the

---

printed 1970). The traditional, usually religious setting and goal for drug consumption are contrasted with present-day laicized use of mind-altering substances.

[113]Charles Levinson, *Valium zum Beispiel: Die multinationalen Konzerne der pharmazeutischen Industrie* (Hamburg: Rowohlt, 1974). The prices charged in India by Glaxo, Pfizer, Hoechst, CIBA-Geigy, and Hoffmann-LaRoche are on the average 357% higher than those listed in the Western countries where these firms have their home offices.

[114]See also Burack, *New Handbook of Prescription Drugs.*

[115]In most countries, most information on drugs for the physician comes from industry-sponsored manuals such as *Physicians' Desk Reference to Pharmaceutical Specialties and Biologicals,* published since 1946 by Medical Economics, Rutherford, N.J. This annual publication, known as *PDR,* is supported by the pharmaceutical industry. The drug descriptions are written by the companies themselves, which pay $115 per column-inch for the space; see John Pekkanen, *The American Connection: Profiteering and Politicking in the "Ethical" Drug Industry* (Chicago: Follett, 1973), p. 106. The French *Vidal* contains descriptions which suppress the warnings that are obligatory in the leaflet that comes with the drug. In contrast to these, the U.S. has two semiofficial pharmacological compendia, the *Pharmacopeia of the United States of America* (*USP*) and the *National Formulary* (*NF*). The *USP* has consistent-

"instrumental consumer," the doctor who prescribes but does not pay for the product. To promote Valium, Hoffmann-LaRoche spent $200 million in ten years and commissioned some two hundred doctors a year to produce scientific articles about its properties.[116] In 1973, the entire drug industry spent an average of $4,500 on each practicing physician for advertising and promotion, about the equivalent of the cost of a year in medical school; in the same year, the industry contributed less than 3 percent to the budget of American medical schools.[117]

Surprisingly, however, the per capita use of medically prescribed drugs around the world seems to have little to do with commercial promotion; it correlates mostly with the number of doctors, even in socialist countries where the education of physicians is not influenced by drug industry publicity and where corporate drug-pushing is limited.[118] Over-all drug consumption in industrial societies is not fundamentally affected by the proportion of items sold by

---

ly given consideration to therapeutic worth and toxicity. These compendia are *not* written for the guidance of physicians, but to provide drug manufacturers with technical standards that preparations must meet to be marketed legally in interstate commerce in the U.S.

[116]For an idea of the number of physicians at the service of a single manufacturer in the decision to promote just one product consult *Librium: Worldwide Bibliography,* published yearly since 1959 by Roche Laboratories. The first four years contain 832 entries. See also *Science* 180 (1973): 1038, for a report of a study conducted by the Federal Drug Administration on the ethics of physicians who conduct field research with new drugs. One-fifth of those investigated had invented the data they sent to the drug companies, and pocketed the fees.

[117]Selig Greenberg, *The Quality of Mercy: A Report on the Critical Condition of Hospital and Medical Care in America* (New York: Atheneum, 1971).

[118]H. Friebel, "Arzneimittelverbrauchs-Studien," in H. J. Dengler and W. Wirth, eds., *Seminar für Klinische Pharmakologie auf Schloss Reisenberg bie Günzburg/Donau, vom 25.–29. Oktober, 1971,* Überreicht von der Medizinisch-Pharmazeutischen Studiengesellschaft E.V., Frankfurt am Main, pp. 228–40. Short, valuable statement on the lack of useful measurements, which makes such a broad statement the best that can be responsibly offered. The author is a director of the Drug Efficacy and Safety Division of the World Health Organization.

prescription, over the counter, or illegally, and it is not affected by whether the purchase is paid for out of pocket, through prepaid insurance, or through welfare funds.[119] In all countries, doctors work increasingly with two groups of addicts: those for whom they prescribe drugs, and those who suffer from their consequences. The richer the community, the larger the percentage of patients who belong to both.[120]

To blame the drug industry for prescribed-drug addiction is therefore as irrelevant as blaming the Mafia[121] for the use of illicit drugs. The current pattern of overconsumption of drugs—be they effective remedy or anodyne; prescription item or part of everyday diet; free, for sale, or stolen—can be explained only as the result of a belief that so far has developed in every culture where the market for consumer goods has reached a critical volume. This pattern is consistent with the ideology of any society oriented towards open-ended enrichment, regardless whether its industrial product is meant for distribution by the presumption of planners or by the forces of the market. In such a society, people come to believe that in health care, as in all other fields of endeavor, technology can be used to change the human condition

---

[119]World Health Organization, Regional Office for Europe, *Consumption of Drugs: Report on a Symposium, Oslo, November 3–7, 1969.* Limited edition, available only to persons with official professional standing through the WHO regional office in Copenhagen. This study is the first of its kind. It compares 22 countries, noting significant differences in drug-consumption patterns but enormous difficulties in establishing precise comparisons. Therapeutic categories, cost evaluations, and measurements for pharmacological units differ. From the information it is legitimate to deduce that total consumption of medicine is largely independent of cost or of the kind of practice that is prevalent, i.e., private or socialized. The consumption in a given country of those drugs that require a prescription is positively related to the density of prescribing physicians.

[120]Alfred M. Freedman, "Drugs and Society: An Ecological Approach," *Comprehensive Psychiatry* 13 (September–October 1972): 411–20.

[121]Alvin Moscow, *Merchants of Heroin* (New York: Dial Press, 1968). This can serve as an introduction to one branch of underworld business.

according to almost any design. Penicillin and DDT, consequently, are viewed as the hors d'oeuvres preceding an era of free lunches. The sickness resulting from each successive course of miracle foods is dealt with by serving still another course of drugs. Thus overconsumption reflects a socially sanctioned, sentimental hankering for yesterday's progress.

The age of new drugs began with aspirin in 1899. Before that time, the doctor himself was without dispute the most important therapeutic agent.[122] Besides opium, the only substances of wide application which would have passed tests for safety and effectiveness were smallpox vaccine, quinine for malaria, and ipecac for dysentery. After 1899 the flood of new drugs continued to rise for half a century. Few of these turned out to be safer, more effective, and cheaper than well-known and long-tested therapeutic standbys, whose numbers grew at a much slower rate. In 1962, when the United States Food and Drug Administration began to examine the 4,300 prescription drugs that had appeared since World War II, only 2 out of 5 were found effective. Many of the new drugs were dangerous, and among those that met FDA standards, few were demonstrably better than those they were meant to replace.[123] Fewer than 98 percent of these chemical substances constitute valuable contributions to the pharmacopeia used in primary care. They include some new kinds of remedies such as antibiotics, but also old remedies which, in the course of the drug age, came to be understood

[122]For the history of the conscious use of the placebo effect, see Arthur K. Shapiro, "A Contribution to a History of the Placebo Effect," *Behavioral Science* 5 (April 1960): 109–35; Gerhard Kienle, *Arzneimittelsicherheit und Gesellschaft: Eine kritische Untersuchung* (Stuttgart: Schattauer, 1974). The ability of the placebo to provoke symptoms of a specific kind, even when given in a double-blind situation, is discussed by Kienle in chap. 7. A mine of international literature on drug safety.

[123]See the statements by Henry Simmons, director of the Food and Drug Administration's Bureau of Drugs, in Nicholas Wade, "Drug Regulation: Food and Drug Administration Replies to Charges by Economists and Industry," *Science* 179 (1973): 775–7.

well enough to be used effectively: digitalis, reserpine, and belladonna are examples. Opinions vary about the actual number of useful drugs: some experienced clinicians believe that less than two dozen basic drugs are all that will ever be desirable for 99 percent of the total population; others, that up to four dozen items are optimal for 98 percent.

The age of great discoveries in pharmacology lies behind us. According to the present director of FDA, the drug age began to decline in 1956. Genuinely new drugs have appeared in decreasing numbers, and many which temporarily glittered in Germany, England, or France, where standards are less stringent than in the United States, Sweden, and Canada, were soon forgotten or are remembered with embarrassment.[124] There is not much territory left to explore. Novelties are either "package deals"—fixed-dose combinations—or medical "me-toos"[125] that are prescribed by physicians because they have been well promoted.[126] The seventeen-year protection that the patent law gives to significant newcomers has run out for most. Now anyone can make them, so long as he does not use the original brand names, which are indefinitely protected by trademark laws. Considerable research has so far produced no reason to suspect that drugs marketed under their generic names in the United States are less effective than their brand-named counterparts, which cost from 3 to 15 times more.[127]

---

[124]*Ibid.*

[125]Fuchs, *Who Shall Live?*

[126]William M. Wardell, "British Usage and American Awareness of Some New Therapeutic Drugs," *Clinical Pharmacology and Therapeutics* 14 (November-December 1973): 1022–34. Studies new drugs which became available in England and were widely discussed in the literature to which U.S. doctors subscribe. Wardell finds that the American specialist is not aware of the existence of these drugs unless they are marketed in the U.S. and that he is therefore subject to enlightenment by detail men.

[127]Medizinisch-Pharmazeutischen Studiengesellschaft E.V., *Bioverfügbarkeit von Arzneistoffen,* Schriftenreihe der Medizinisch-Pharmazeutischen Studiengesellschaft E.V., vol. 6 (Frankfurt:

The fallacy that society is caught forever in the drug age is one of the dogmas with which medical policy-making has been encumbered: it fits industrialized man.[128] He has learned to try to *purchase* whatever he fancies. He gets nowhere without transportation or education; his environment has made it impossible for him to walk, to learn, and to feel in control of his body. To take a drug, no matter which and for what reason—is a last chance to assert control over himself, to interfere on his own with his body rather than let others interfere. The pharmaceutical invasion leads him to medication, by himself or by others, that reduces his ability to cope with a body for which he can still care.

Diagnostic Imperialism

In a medicalized society the influence of physicians extends not only to the purse and the medicine

---

Umschau, 1974). Joint public-relations campaigns conducted by otherwise competing firms deserve special attention. At present, they focus on extolling the superiority of trademarked products over generic equivalents—e.g., of Bayer Aspirin over the generic drug aspirin—on the grounds of "bio-availability," a higher and more controlled biological availability of the drug once it is incorporated into the organism. For any unprejudiced mind, ten years' research has proved that with the one exception of a generic preparation of chloramphenicol (see Burack, *A New Handbook of Prescription Drugs,* p. 85), generic drugs are in no way inferior to those produced under trade names. This conclusion has been incorporated into U.S. federal policy-making. Nevertheless, for the last 5 years the drug companies have sponsored several hundred "research papers" per year on differences in "bio-availability," spending on the author of each paper an average of $6,000 in honoraria, expenses, and costs of attending professional conferences. Many of these authors are department heads of major universities. The conclusions of most papers show no medically significant difference. But the total impact of this phantom research is the mystification of the prescribing general practitioner, who will often recommend the drug advertised for its high "bio-availability," irrespective of its cost.

[128] J. P. Dupuy and A. Letourmy, *Déterminants et coûts sociaux de l'innovation en matière de santé,* report by the OCDE, 1974. The authors support this thesis. The refinement of those criteria by which a specialist measures the effectiveness of his specialized intervention, after a certain threshold, will ensure the appearance of generically predictable unwanted side-effects. If, in their turn, the specific diagnosis and treatment of these side-effects were attempted, this further medical intervention would only reinforce iatrogenesis.

chest but also to the categories to which people are assigned. Medical bureaucrats subdivide people into those who may drive a car, those who may stay away from work, those who must be locked up, those who may become soldiers, those who may cross borders, cook, or practice prostitution,[129] those who may not run for the vice-presidency of the United States, those who are dead,[130] those who are competent to commit a crime, and those who are liable to commit one. On November 5, 1766, the Empress Maria Theresa issued an edict requesting the court physician to certify fitness to undergo torture so as to ensure healthy, i.e. "accurate," testimony; it was one of the first laws to establish mandatory medical certification. Ever since, filling out forms and signing statements have taken up increasingly more medical time.[131] Each kind of certificate provides the holder with a special status based on medical rather than civic opinion.[132] Used outside the therapeutic process, this medicalized status does two obvious things: (1) it exempts the holder from work, prison, military service, or the marriage bond, and (2) it gives others the right to encroach upon the holder's freedom by putting him into an institution or denying him work. In addition, the proliferation of medical

---

[129]On the certification of prostitutes, see William W. Sanger, *The History of Prostitution* (New York: American Medical Press, 1858).

[130]For history of medical death certificates, see U.S. National Office of Vital Statistics, *First Things and Last: The Story of Birth and Death Certificates,* U.S. Public Health Service Publication no. 724 (Washington, D.C., 1960).

[131]Office of Health Economics, *Off Sick,* January 1971, p. 17. It is estimated that between 15 and 30% of all visits to the doctor have no other purpose than obtaining a certificate. In 58% of the cases, the final day of incapacity noted on certificates justifying sick leave is Saturday.

[132]The encroachment of expertise on the rule against hearsay is of course not limited to medicine. It is a common feature of secularization and of the rise of the professions. Inside and outside the courtroom, it whittles away confidence in what the common man sees and hears, and thus undermines both the judicial and the political process. On the author's view of professional expropriation of language, science, and legal procedures, see Ivan Illich, *Tools for Conviviality* (New York: Harper & Row, 1973), pp. 85–99.

certifications can invest school, employment, and politics with opportunities for new therapeutic functions. In a society in which most people are certified as deviants, the milieu for such deviant majorities will come to resemble a hospital. To spend one's life in a hospital is obviously bad for health.

Once a society is so organized that medicine can transform people into patients because they are unborn, newborn, menopausal, or at some other "age of risk," the population inevitably loses some of its autonomy to its healers. The ritualization of stages in life is nothing new;[133] what is new is their intense medicalization. The sorcerer or medicine man—as opposed to the malevolent witch—dramatized the progress of an Azandé tribesman from one stage of his health to the next.[134] The experience may have been painful,[135] but the ritual was short and it served society in highlighting its own regenerative powers.[136] Lifelong medical supervision is something else. It turns life into a series of periods of risk, each calling for tutelage of a special kind. From the crib to the office and from the Club Mediterranée to the terminal ward, each age-cohort is conditioned by a

---

[133] Franz Boll, "Die Lebensalter: Ein Beitrag zur antiken Ethologie und zur Geschichte der Zahlen," *Neue Jahrbücher für das klassische Altertum, Geschichte und deutsche Literatur* 16, no. 31 (1913): 89–145.

[134] See E. E. Evans-Pritchard, *Witchcraft, Oracles, and Magic Among the Azandé* (New York: Oxford Univ. Press, 1937), for the distinction of the sorcerer from the witch. This distinction is refined and applied to Western culture by Jeffrey B. Russell, *Witchcraft in the Middle Ages* (Ithaca, N.Y.: Cornell Univ. Press, 1972). The demonological element that transforms the sorceress into a heretic is usually grafted on at the level of the courts.

[135] Victor W. Turner, "Betwixt and Between: The Liminal Period in *Rites de Passage*," in American Ethnological Society, *Symposium on New Approaches to the Study of Religion: Proceedings, 1964* (Seattle: Univ. of Washington Press, 1965), pp. 4–20. By medicalization of life, what appeared to be "liminal" in past societies has been made the everyday situation of administered man.

[136] Arnold van Gennep, *The Rites of Passage* (London: Routledge, 1960 [French original, 1909]). The recent critique of the author by Lévy-Strauss has not called into question his basic idea that periods of initiation affirm and symbolize the continuing health-maintaining function of culture.

milieu that defines health for those whom it segregates. Hygenic bureaucracy stops the parent in front of the school and the minor in front of the court, and takes the old out of the home. By becoming a specialized place, school, work, or home is made unfit for most people. The hospital, the modern cathedral, lords it over this hieratic environment of health devotees. From Stockholm to Wichita the towers of the medical center impress on the landscape the promise of a conspicuous final embrace. For rich and poor, life is turned into a pilgrimage through check-ups and clinics back to the ward where it started.[137] Life is thus reduced to a "span," to a statistical phenomenon which, for better or for worse, must be institutionally planned and shaped. This life-span is brought into existence with the prenatal check-up, when the doctor decides if and how the fetus shall be born, and it will end with a mark on a chart ordering resuscitation suspended. Between delivery and termination this bundle of biomedical care fits best into a city that is built like a mechanical womb. At each stage of their lives people are age-specifically disabled. The old are the most obvious example: they are victims of treatments meted out for an incurable condition.[138]

---

[137]For literature on the subtle penetration of the hospital into the interstices of the modern city consult Gerald F. Pyle. "The Geography of Health Care," in John Melton Hunter, *The Geography of Health and Disease,* Studies in Geography no. 6 (Chapel Hill, N.C.: Univ. of North Carolina Press, 1974), a spatial analysis at the service of health planners. For a book-length treatment of the architectonic impact of hospitals on our society, see Roslyn Lindheim, *The Hospitalization of Space* (London: Calder & Boyars, 1976). Lindheim demonstrates how the reorganization of spatial patterns at the service of physicians has impoverished the nonmedical, health-supporting, and healing aspects of the social and physical environment for modern man.

[138]For orientation on the social science literature on the old and aging, see James E. Birren, Yonina Talmon and Earl F. Cheit, "Aging: 1. Psychological Aspects; 2. Social Aspects; 3. Economic Aspects," *International Encyclopedia of the Social Sciences* (1968), 1:176–202. For orientation on German literature, see Volkmar Boehlau, ed., *Wege zur Erforschung des Alterns,* Wege der Forschung, vol. 189 (Darmstadt: Wissenschaftliche Buchgesellschaft, 1973), an anthology. On French contemporary aging, Michel Philibert, *L'Échelle des âges* (Paris: Seuil, 1968).

Most of man's ailments consist of illnesses that are acute and benign—either self-limiting or subject to control through a few dozen routine interventions.[139] For a wide range of conditions, those who are treated least probably make the best progress. "For the sick," Hippocrates said, "the least is best." More often than not, the best a learned and conscientious physician can do is convince his patient that he can live with his impairment, reassure him of an eventual recovery or of the availability of morphine at the time when he will need it, do for him what grandmother could have done, and otherwise defer to nature.[140] The new tricks that have frequent application are so simple that the last generation of grandmothers would have learned them long ago had they not been browbeaten into incompetency by medical mystification. Boy-scout training, good-Samaritan laws, and the duty to carry first-aid equipment in each car would prevent more highway deaths than any fleet of helicopter-ambulances. Those other interventions which are part of primary care and which, though they require the work of specialists, have been proved effective on a population basis can be employed more effectively if my neighbor or I feel responsible for recognizing when they are needed and applying first treatment. For acute sickness, treatment so complex that it requires a specialist is often ineffective and much more often inaccessible or simply too late. After twenty years of socialized medicine in England and Wales, doctors get to coronary cases on an average of four hours after the beginning of symptoms, and by this time 50 percent of patients are

---

[139]John H. Dingle, "The Ills of Man," *Scientific American* 229 (September 1973): 77–82. The study that comes to this "conclusion" is broadly based. It distinguishes four perspectives on "ailment": (1) people, (2) physicians, (3) patients, (4) compilers of vital statistics. From all four points of view this conclusion seems to hold.

[140]Max Neuburger, *The Doctrine of the Healing Power of Nature Throughout the Course of Time*, trans. L. J. Boyd (New York: privately printed, 1932). For more recent references, Joseph Schumacher, *Antike Medizin: Die naturphilosophischen Grundlagen der Medizin in der griechischen Antike* (Berlin: Gruyter, 1963).

dead.[141] The fact that modern medicine has become very effective in the treatment of specific symptoms does not mean that it has become more beneficial for the health of the patient.

With some qualifications, the severe limits of effective medical treatment apply not only to conditions that have long been recognized as sickness—rheumatism, appendicitis, heart failure, degenerative disease, and many infectious diseases—but even more drastically to those that have only recently generated demands for medical care. Old age, for example, which has been variously considered a doubtful privilege or a pitiful ending but never a disease,[142] has recently been put under doctor's orders. The demand for old-age care has increased, not just because there are more old people who survive, but also because there are more people who state their claim that their old age should be cured.

The maximum life-span has not changed, but the average life-span has. Life expectancy at birth has increased enormously. Many more children survive, no matter how sickly and in need of a special environment and special care. The life expectancy of young adults is still increasing in some poorer countries. But in rich countries the life expectancy of those between fifteen and forty-five has tended to stabilize because accidents[143] and the new diseases of civilization kill as many as formerly succumbed to pneumonia and other infections. Relatively more old people are around, and they are increasingly prone to be ill, out

---

[141]J. F. Partridge and J. S. Geddes, "A Mobile Intensive-Care Unit in the Management of Myocardial Infarction," *Lancet,* 1967, 2:271.

[142]Simone de Beauvoir, *The Coming of Age: The Study of the Aging Process,* trans. Patrick O'Brian (New York: Putnam, 1972). A monumental treatment of old age throughout history in the perspective of contemporary aging. See also Jean Amery, *Über das Alter: Revolte und Resignation* (Stuttgart: Klette, 1968), an exceptionally sensitive contemporary phenomenology of aging.

[143]*World Health Statistics Report* 27, September 1974. An international comparison of 27 industrialized countries shows that for the age group 15–44 years old, accidents were the leading cause of death in 1971 (except for England and Wales). In half of these countries they accounted for more than 30% of all deaths.

of place, and helpless. No matter how much medicine they take, no matter what care is given them, a life expectancy of sixty-five years has remained unchanged over the past century. Medicine just cannot do much for the illness associated with aging, and even less about the process and experience of aging itself.[144] It cannot cure cardiovascular disease, most cancers, arthritis, advanced cirrhosis, not even the common cold. It is fortunate that some of the pain the aged suffer can be lessened. Unfortunately, though, most treatment of the old requiring professional intervention not only tends to heighten their pain but, if successful, also to protract it.[145]

Old age has been medicalized at precisely the historical moment when it has become a more common occurrence for demographic reasons; 28 percent of the American medical budget is spent on the 10 percent of the population who are over sixty five. This minority is outgrowing the remainder of the population at an annual rate of 3 percent, while the per capita cost of their care is rising 5 to 7 percent faster than the over-all per capita cost. As more of the elderly acquire rights to professional care, opportunities for independent aging decline. More have to seek refuge in institutions. Simultaneously, as more of the elderly are initiated into treatment for the correction of incorrigible impairment or for the cure of incurable disease, the number of unmet claims for old-age services snowballs.[146] If the eyesight of an old woman fails, her plight will not be recognized unless she en-

---

[144]David Jutman, "The Hunger of Old Men," *Trans-Action*, November 12, 1971, pp. 55–66.

[145]A. N. Exton-Smith, "Terminal Illness in the Aged," *Lancet*, 1961, 2:305–8. Most pain and suffering are associated with processes that lead indirectly to death. Although the use of antibiotics may avert or delay complications such as bronchopneumonia, which would otherwise be fatal, this often adds little time and much pain to a life.

[146]Rick Carlson, in *The End of Medicine* (New York: Wiley Interscience, 1975), develops this whole point very well. See also H. Harmsen, "Die sozialmedizinische Bedeutung der Erhöhung der Lebenserwartung und der Zunahme des Anteils der Bejahrten bis 1980," *Physikalische Medizin und Rehabilitation* 9, no. 5 (1968): 119–21.

ters the "blindness establishment"—one of the eight hundred-odd United States agencies which produce services for the blind, preferably for the young and those who can be rehabilitated for work.[147] Since she is neither young nor of working age, she will receive only a grudging welcome; at the same time, she will have difficulty fitting into the old-age establishment. She will thus be marginally medicalized by two sets of institutions, the one designed to socialize her among the blind, the other to medicalize her decrepitude.

As more old people become dependent on professional services, more people are pushed into specialized institutions for the old, while the home neighborhood becomes increasingly inhospitable to those who hang on.[148] These institutions seem to be the contemporary strategy for the disposal of the old, who have been institutionalized in more frank and arguably less hideous forms by most other societies.[149] The mortality rate during the first year after institutionalization is significantly higher than the rate for those who stay in their accustomed surroundings.[150] Separation from home contributes to the appearance and mortality of many a serious dis-

---

[147]Robert A. Scott, *The Making of Blind Men* (New York: Russell Sage, 1969). Being accepted among the blind and behaving like a blind person are to a great extent independent of the degree of optical impairment. For most of the "blind," it is above all the result of their successful client relationship to an agency concerned with "blindness."

[148]Roslyn Lindheim, "Environments for the Elderly: Future-Oriented Design for Living?" February 20, 1974, mimeographed. Describes the way the old experience space.

[149]On the social elimination of the old the main source remains John Koty, *Die Behandlung der Alten und Kranken bei den Naturvölkern* (Stuttgart: Hirschfeld, 1934). I have not seen Fritz Paudler, *Die Alten- und Krankentötung als Sitte bei den indogermanischen Völkern* (Heidelberg, 1936). Complete reference to the literature in Will-Eich Peuckert, ed., "Altentötung," in *Handwörterbuch der Sage* (Göttingen: Vandenhoeck & Ruprecht, 1961).

[150]A. Jores and H. G. Puchta, "Der Pensionierungstod: Untersuchungen an Hamburger Beamten," *Medizinische Klinik* 54, no. 25 (1959): 1158–64.

ease.[151] Some old people seek institutionalization with the intention of shortening their lives.[152] Dependence is always painful, and more so for the old. Privilege or poverty in earlier life reaches a climax in modern old age. Only the very rich and the very independent can choose to avoid that medicalization of the end to which the poor must submit and which becomes increasingly intense and universal as the society they live in becomes richer.[153] The transformation of old age into a condition calling for professional services has cast the elderly in the role of a minority who will feel painfully deprived at any relative level of tax-supported privilege. From weak old people who are sometimes miserable and bitterly disappointed by neglect, they are turned into certified

---

[151] David Bakan, *Disease, Pain and Sacrifice: Toward a Psychology of Suffering* (Boston: Beacon Press, 1971). These diseases include asthma, cancer, congestive heart failure, diabetes mellitus, disseminated lupus, functional uterine bleeding, Raynaud's disease, rheumatoid arthritis, thyrotoxicosis, tuberculosis and ulcerative colitis. See *ibid.* for literature on each.

[152] Elisabeth Markson, "A Hiding Place To Die," *Trans-Action*, November 12, 1972, pp. 48–54. A pathetic and sensitive report. See also Jutman, "The Hunger of Old Men." The old have always obliged by dying on request: David Lester, "Voodoo Death: Some New Thoughts on an Old Phenomenon," *American Anthropologist* 74 (June 1972): 386–90; Walter B. Cannon, "Voodoo Death," *American Anthropologist* 44 (April–June 1942): 169–81. There were always ways of driving them to suicide: J. Wisse, *Selbstmord und Todesfurcht bei den Naturvölkern* (Zutphen: Thieme, 1933). Margaret Blenkner, et al. "Protective services for older people." Findings from the Benjamin Rose Institute Study, final report. Cleveland, Rose Institute, 1974. Professional home-aid, though representing the "best" social work thinking and practice also tends to accelerate the decline and death of the old when it goes beyond simple house-cleaning, garbage removal and home repair. Two years after the onset of *intensive* home-care delivery, 39% of the assisted were dead, as compared with only 25% in the randomly selected control group.

[153] Peter Townsend, *The Last Refuge: A Survey of Residential Institutions and Homes for the Aged in England and Wales* (London: Routledge, 1962). Complements previous work done by the author. Evaluates residential accommodations as provided under the British National Assistance Act of 1948 and points to the lack of equity in treatment. Anne-Marie Guillemard, *La Retraite, une mort sociale: Sociologie des conduites en situation de retraite* (Paris: Mouton, 1972). A socio-economic study which shows that class discrimination is strongly accentuated in French retirement.

members of the saddest of consumer groups, that of the aged programmed never to get enough.[154] What medical labeling has done to the end of life, it has equally done to its beginning. Just as the doctor's power was first affirmed over old age and eventually encroached on early retirement and climacteric, so his authority over the delivery room, which dates from the mid-nineteenth century, spread to the nursery, the kindergarten, and the classroom and medicalized infancy, childhood, and puberty. But while it has become acceptable to advocate limits to the escalation of costly care for the old, limits to so-called medical investments in childhood are still a subject that seems taboo. Industrial parents, forced to procreate manpower for a world into which nobody fits who has not been crushed and molded by sixteen years of formal education, feel impotent to care personally for their offspring and, in despair, shower them with medicine.[155] Proposals to reduce medical outputs in the United States from their present level of about $100 billion to their 1950 level of $10 billion, or to close medical schools in Colombia, never turn into controversial issues because those who make them are soon discredited as heartless proponents of infanticide or of mass extermination of the poor. The engineering approach to the making of economically productive adults has made death in childhood a scandal, impairment through early disease a public embarrassment, unrepaired congenital malformation an intolerable sight, and the possibility of eugenic birth control a preferred theme for international congresses in the seventies.

As for infant mortality, it has indeed been re-

---

[154]A. Eardley and J. Wakefield, *What Patients Think About the Christie Hospital,* University Hospital of South Manchester, 1974. From year to year the demands made by people at a certain age above 70 become more specific and costly.

[155]The "baby" is a rather recently developed social category: the first stage in the development of man-the-consumer. On the process by which the suckling was slowly turned into a baby and the assistance that medicine provided in this process, see Luc Boltanski, "Prime education et morale de classe," *Cahiers du Centre de sociologie européenne* (The Hague/Paris: Mouton, 1969).

duced. Life expectancy in the developed countries has increased from thirty-five years in the eighteenth century to seventy years today. This is due mainly to the reduction of infant mortality in these countries; for example, in England and Wales the number of infant deaths per 1,000 live births declined from 154 in 1840 to 22 in 1960. But it would be entirely incorrect to attribute more than one of those lives "saved" to a curative intervention that presupposes anything like a doctor's training, and it would be a delusion to attribute the infant mortality rate of poor countries, which in some cases is ten times that of the United States, to a lack of doctors. Food, antisepsis, civil engineering, and above all, a new widespread disvalue placed on the death of a child,[156] no matter how weak or malformed, are much more significant factors and represent changes that are only remotely related to medical intervention. While in gross infant mortality the United States ranks seventeenth among nations, infant mortality among the poor is much higher than among higher-income groups. In New York City, infant mortality among the black population is more than twice as high as for the population in general, and probably higher than in many underdeveloped areas such as Thailand and Jamaica.[157] The insistence that more doctors are needed to prevent infants from dying can thus be understood as a way of avoiding income equalization while at the same time creating more jobs for professionals. It

---

[156]The culture of childhood as that characteristic for an age group distinct from the adult and the infant is of social origin, like that of the "baby." See Philippe Ariés, *Centuries of Childhood: A Social History of Family Life* (New York: Knopf, 1962), especially on the profound change the attitude towards the death of a child underwent between the 17th and the 19th centuries. Suse Barth, Lebensalter-Darstellungen im 19 and 20. Jahrhundert. Ikonographische Studie. Inauguraldissertation, Ludwig-Maximilian Universitaet, Muenchen, 1971. Akademischer Photodruck, Bamberg. The iconography of the "child" during the 19th and 20th centuries. Only in this period are the "ages of man" symbolized by references to one class only, namely the bourgeoisie, and are perceived as "psychological problems."

[157]John Bryant, M.D., *Health and the Developing World* (Ithaca, N.Y.: Cornell Univ. Press, 1969).

would be equally reckless to claim that those changes in the general environment that do have a causal relationship to the presence of doctors represent a positive balance for health. Although physicians did pioneer antisepsis, immunization, and dietary supplements, they were also involved in the switch to the bottle that transformed the traditional suckling into a modern baby and provided industry with working mothers who are clients for a factory-made formula.

The damage this switch does to natural immunity mechanisms fostered by human milk and the physical and emotional stress caused by bottle feeding are comparable to if not greater than the benefits that a population can derive from specific immunizations.[158] Even more serious is the contribution the bottle makes to the menace of worldwide protein starvation. For instance, in 1960, 96 percent of Chilean mothers breast-fed their infants up to and beyond the first birthday. Then, for a decade, Chilean women underwent intense political indoctrination by both right-wing Christian Democrats and a variety of left-wing parties. By 1970 only 6 percent breast-fed beyond the first year and 80 percent had weaned their infants before the second full month. As a result, 84 percent of potential human breast milk now remains unproduced. The milk of an additional 32,000 cows would have to be added to Chile's overgrazed pastures to compensate—as far as possible—for this loss.[159] As the bottle became a status symbol, new illnesses

---

[158]About the relatively much higher resistánce to malaria, infections, and deficiency diseases of breast-fed babies, see "Milk and Malaria," *British Medical Journal,* 1952, 2:1405, and 1953, 2:1210. O. Mellander and B. Vahlquiest, "Breast Feeding and Artificial Feeding," *Acta Paediatrica* 2, suppl. (1958): 101. For a survey of literature, the editorial "Breast Feeding and Polio Susceptibility," *Nutrition Review,* May 1965, pp. 131–3. Leonardo J. Mata and Richard Wyatt, "Host Resistance to Infection," *American Journal of Clinical Nutrition* 24 (August 1971): 976–86.

[159]For more data on the impact of the bottle on world nutrition, see Alan Berg, *The Nutrition Factor: Its Role in National Development* (Washington, D.C.: Brookings Institution, 1973). A child nursed through the first two years of its life receives the nutritional equivalent of 461 quarts of cow's milk, which costs the equivalent of the average yearly income of an Indian.

appeared among children who had been denied the breast, and since mothers lack traditional know-how to deal with babies who do not behave like sucklings, babies became new consumers of medical attention and of its risks.[160] The sum total of physical impairment due just to this substitution of marketed baby food for mother's milk is difficult to balance against the benefits derived from curative medical intervention in childhood sickness and from surgical correction of birth defects ranging from harelip to heart defects.

It can, of course, be argued that the medical classification of age groups according to their diagnosed need for health commodities does not generate ill-health but only reflects the health-denying breakdown of the family as a cocoon, of the neighborhood as a network of gift relationships, and of the environment as the shelter of a local subsistence community. No doubt, it is true that a medicalized social perception reflects a reality that is determined by the organization of capital-intensive production, and that it is the corresponding social pattern of nuclear families, welfare agencies, and polluted nature that degrades home, neighborhood, and milieu. But medicine does not simply mirror reality; it reinforces and reproduces the process that undermines the social cocoons within which man has evolved. Medical classification justifies the imperialism of standard staples like baby food over mother's milk and of old-age homes over a corner at home. By turning the newborn into a hospitalized patient until he or she is certified as healthy, and by defining grandmother's complaint as a need for treatment rather than for patient respect, the medical enterprise creates not only biologically formulated legitimacy for man-the-consumer but also new pressures for an escalation of the megama-

[160]The pattern of worldwide modern malnutrition is reflected in the two forms that infant malnutrition takes. The switch from the breast to the bottle introduces Chilean babies to a life of endemic undernourishment; the same switch initiates British babies into a life of sickening, addictive overalimentation: see R. K. Oates, "Infant Feeding Practices," *British Medical Journal,* 1973, 2:762–4.

chine.[161] Genetic selection of those who fit into that machine is the logical next step of medicosocial control.

Preventive Stigma

As curative treatment focuses increasingly on conditions in which it is ineffectual, expensive, and painful, medicine has begun to market prevention. The concept of morbidity has been enlarged to cover prognosticated risks. Along with sick-care, health care has become a commodity, something one pays for rather than something one does. The higher the salary the company pays, the higher the rank of an *aparatchik,* the more will be spent to keep the valuable cog well oiled. Maintenance costs for highly capitalized manpower are the new measure of status for those on the upper rungs. People keep up with the Joneses by emulating their "check-ups," an English word which has entered French, Serbian, Spanish, Malay, and Hungarian dictionaries. People are turned into patients without being sick. The medicalization of prevention thus becomes another major symptom of social iatrogenesis. It tends to transform personal responsibility for my future into my management by some agency.

Usually the danger of routine diagnosis is even less feared than the danger of routine treatment, though social, physical, and psychological torts inflicted by medical classification are no less well documented. Diagnoses made by the physician and his helpers can define either temporary or permanent roles for the patient. In either case, they add to a biophysical condition a social state created by presumably authoritative evaluation.[162] When a veteri-

---

[161]On life as a constant training for survival in the megamachine, see Lewis Mumford, *The Pentagon of Power: The Myth of the Machine, Volume 2* (New York: Harcourt Brace, 1970).

[162]Thomas J. Scheff, *Being Mentally Ill: A Sociological Theory* (Chicago: Aldine, 1966). Though he deals primarily with psychiatric issues, Scheff does stress the analytic difference between mental illness that is part of the social system and the corresponding behavior.

narian diagnoses a cow's distemper, it doesn't usually affect the patient's behavior. When a doctor diagnoses a human being, it does.[163] In those instances where the physician functions as healer he confers on the person recognized as sick certain rights, duties, and excuses which have a conditional and temporary legitimacy and which lapse when the patient is healed; most sickness leaves no taint of deviance or disorderly conduct on the patient's reputation. No one is interested in ex-allergics or ex-appendectomy patients, just as no one will be remembered as an ex-traffic offender. In other instances, however, the physician acts primarily as an actuary, and his diagnosis can defame the patient, and sometimes his children, for life. By attaching irreversible degradation to a person's identity, it brands him forever with a permanent stigma.[164] The objective condition may have long since disappeared, but the iatrogenic label sticks. Like ex-convicts, former mental patients, people after their first heart attack, former alcoholics, carriers of the sickle-cell trait, and (until recently) ex-tuberculotics are transformed into outsiders for the rest of their lives. Professional suspicion alone is enough to legitimize the stigma even if the suspected condition never existed. The medical label may protect the patient from punishment only to submit him to interminable instruction, treatment, and discrimination, which are inflicted on him for his professionally presumed benefit.[165]

In the past, medicine labeled people in two

---

[163]Freidson, *Profession of Medicine*, p. 223.

[164]Erving Goffman, *Stigma: Notes on the Management of Spoiled Identity* (Englewood Cliffs, N.J.: Spectrum 1963). See also Richard Sennett, "Two on the Aisle," *New York Review of Books*, November 1, 1973, who underlines that for Goffman the central task is a description of the consciousness induced by living in a modern city. Contemporary life inevitably stigmatizes; on the mechanisms see H. P. Dreitzel, *Die gesellschaftlichen Leiden und das Leiden an der Gesellschaft: Vorstudien zu einer Pathologie des Rollenverhaltens* (Stuttgart: Enke, 1972).

[165]Wilhelm Aubert and Sheldon Messinger, "The Criminal and the Sick," *Inquiry* 1 (1958): 137–60. Discusses the different forms

ways: those for whom cures could be attempted, and those who were beyond repair, such as lepers, cripples, oddities, and the dying. Either way, diagnosis could lead to stigma. Medicalized prevention now creates a third way. It turns the physician into an officially licensed magician whose prophecies cripple even those who are left unharmed by his brews.[166] Diagnosis may exclude a human being with bad genes from being born, another from promotion, and a third from political life. The mass hunt for health risks begins with dragnets designed to apprehend those needing special protection: prenatal medical visits; well-child-care clinics for infants; school and camp check-ups and prepaid medical schemes.[167] Recently genetic and blood pressure "counseling" services were added. The United States proudly led the world in organizing disease-hunts and, later, in questioning their utility.[168]

In the past decade, automated multiphasic health-testing became operational and was welcomed as the poor man's escalator into the world of Mayo and Massachusetts General. This assembly-line procedure of complex chemical and medical examinations can

---

social control can take, depending on the special way in which stigma impinges on moral identity.

[166]Fred Davis, *Passage Through Crisis: Polio Victims and Their Families* (Indianapolis: Bobbs-Merrill, 1963). Davis relates transitoriness not only to seriousness but also to social class. The poor will be diagnosed as "permanently impaired" much sooner than the rich.

[167]C. M. Wylie, "Participation in a Multiple Screening Clinic with Five-Year Follow-up," *Public Health Reports* 76 (July 1961): 596–602. Report indicates disappointing results.

[168]G. S. Siegel, "The Uselessness of Periodic Examination," *Archives of Environmental Health* 13 (September 1966): 292–5. "Periodic health examination of adults, as originally conceived and currently practiced, remains, after 50 years of vigorous American promotion, a scientifically unproven medical procedure. We do not have conclusive evidence that a population receiving such care lives longer, better, healthier, or happier because of it, nor do we have evidence to the contrary." Heinrich Schipperges, Aerztliche Bemuehungen um die Gesunderhaltung seit der Antike. in: Heidelberger Jahrbuecher, 7, 1963, p. 121–36. A history of medicalized health-maintenance since antiquity.

be performed by paraprofessional technicians at a surprisingly low cost. It purports to offer uncounted millions more sophisticated detection of hidden therapeutic needs than was available in the sixties even for the most "valuable" hierarchs in Houston or Moscow. At the outset of this testing, the lack of controlled studies allowed the salesmen of mass-produced prevention to foster unsubstantiated expectations. (More recently, controlled comparative studies of population groups benefitting from maintenance service and early diagnosis have become available; two dozen such studies indicate that these diagnostic procedures—even when followed by high-level medical treatments—have no positive impact on life expectancy.[169]) Ironically, the serious asymptomatic disorders which this kind of screening alone can discover among adults are frequently incurable illnesses in which early treatment only aggravates the patient's physical condition. In any case, it transforms people who feel healthy into patients anxious for their verdict.

In the detection of sickness medicine does two things: it "discovers" new disorders, and it ascribes these disorders to concrete individuals. To discover a new category of disease is the pride of the medical scientist.[170] To ascribe the pathology to some Tom, Dick, or Harry is the first task of the physician acting as member of a consulting profession.[171] Trained to "do something" and express his concern, he feels ac-

---

[169] Paul D. Clote, "Automated Multiphasic Health Testing: An Evaluation," independent study with John McKnight, Northwestern University, 1973; reproduced in Antología A8 (Cuernavaca: CIDOC, 1974). Reviews the available literature.

[170] J. Schwartz and G. L. Baum, "The History of Histoplasmosis," *New England Journal of Medicine* 256 (1957): 253–8. Describes the costly discovery of an incurable "disease" that neither kills nor impairs and seems to be endemic wherever people come in contact with chickens, cattle, cats, or dogs.

[171] Freidson, *Profession of Medicine,* pp. 73 ff., makes the distinction I here apply. As a scholarly professional, the medical scientist need contend only with his colleagues and their acceptance of his "invention" of a new disease. As a consulting professional, the practicing physician depends on an educated public that accepts his exclusive right to diagnose.

tive, useful, and effective when he can diagnose disease.[172] Though theoretically, at the first encounter the physician does not presume that his patient is affected by a disease, yet through a form of fail-safe principle he usually acts as if imputing a disease to the patient were better than disregarding one. The medical-decision rule pushes him to seek safety by diagnosing illness rather than health.[173] The classic demonstration of this bias came in an experiment conducted in 1934.[174] In a survey of 1,000 eleven-year-old children from the public schools of New York, 61 percent were found to have had their tonsils removed. "The remaining 39 percent were subjected to examination by a group of physicians, who selected 45 percent of these for tonsillectomy and rejected the rest. The rejected children were re-examined by another group of physicians, who recommended tonsillectomy for 46 percent of those remaining after the first examination. When the rejected children were examined a third time, a similar percentage was selected for tonsillectomy so that after three examinations only sixty-five children remained who had not been recommended for tonsillectomy. These subjects were not further examined because the supply of examining physicians ran out."[175] This test was conducted at a free clinic, where financial considerations could not explain the bias.

Diagnostic bias in favor of sickness combines with frequent diagnostic error. Medicine not only imputes questionable categories with inquisitorial enthusiasm; it does so at a rate of miscarriage that no court system could tolerate. In one instance, autopsies showed that more than half the patients who died in a

---

[172]Parsons, *The Social System*, pp. 466 ff. The author makes this point commenting on Pareto.

[173]Thomas J. Scheff, "Decision Rules, Types of Error, and Their Consequences in Medical Diagnosis," *Behavioral Science* 8 (1963): 97–107.

[174]American Child Health Association, *Physical Defects: The Pathway to Correction* (New York, 1934), chap. 8, pp. 80–96.

[175]Harry Bakwin, "Pseudodoxia Pediatrica," *New England Journal of Medicine* 232 (1945): 691–97.

British university clinic with a diagnosis of specific heart failure had in fact died of something else. In another instance, the same series of chest X-rays shown to the same team of specialists on different occasions led them to change their mind on 20 percent of all cases. Up to three times as many patients will tell Dr. Smith that they cough, produce sputum, or suffer from stomach cramps as will tell Dr. Jones. Up to one-quarter of simple hospital tests show seriously divergent results when done from the same sample in two different labs.[176] Nor do machines seem to be any more infallible. In a competition between diagnostic machines and human diagnosticians in 83 cases recommended for pelvic surgery, pathology showed that both man and machine were correct in 22 instances; in 37 instances the computer correctly rejected the doctor's diagnosis; in 11 instances the doctors proved the computer wrong; and in 10 cases both were in error.[177]

In addition to diagnostic bias and error, there is wanton aggression.[178] A cardiac catheterization, used

---

[176]For references and further bibliography see L. H. Garland, "Studies on the Accuracy of Diagnostic Procedures," *American Journal of Roentgenology, Radium Therapy, and Nuclear Medicine* 82 (July 1959): 25–38. See also A. L. Cochrane and L. H. Garland, "Observer Error in the Interpretation of Chest Films: An International Comparison," *Lancet* 263 (1952): 505–9. Suggests that American diagnosticians might have a stronger penchant for positive findings than their British counterparts. A L. Cochrane, P. J. Chapman, and P. D. Oldham, "Observers' Errors in Taking Medical Histories," *Lancet* 260 (1951): 1007–9.

[177]Osler Peterson, Ernest M. Barsamian, and Murray Eden, "A Study of Diagnostic Performance: A Preliminary Report," *Journal of Medical Education* 41 (August 1966): 797–803.

[178]Maurice Pappworth, *Human Guinea Pigs: Experimentation on Man* (Boston: Beacon Press, 1968). In 1967 Dr. Pappworth published a report on experimental diagnostic procedures that involved high risks of permanent damage or death, which had recently been described in the most respectable medical journals and were often performed on nonpatients, infants, pregnant women, mental defectives, and the old. He has been attacked for rendering a disservice to his profession, for undermining the trust lay people have in doctors, and for publishing in a paperpack what could "ethically" be told only in literature written for doctors. Perhaps most surprising in these reports is the relentless repetition of identical high-risk procedures for the sole purpose of earning academic promotions.

to determine if a patient is suffering from cardiomyopathy—admittedly, this is not done routinely—costs $350 and kills one patient in fifty. Yet there is no evidence that a *differential* diagnosis based on its results extends either the life expectancy or the comfort of the patient.[179] Most tests are less murderous and much more commonly performed, but many still involve known risks to the individual or his offspring which are high enough to obscure the value of whatever information they can provide. Many routine uses of X-rays and fluoroscope on the young, the injection or ingestion of reagents and tracers, and the use of Ritalin to diagnose hyperactivity in children are examples.[180] Attendance in public schools where teachers are vested with delegated medical powers constitutes a major health risk for children.[181] Even

---

[179]"Such a procedure is as informative as recording a patient's blood pressure once in a lifetime, or examining his urine once every 20 years. This practice is ridiculous, absurd and unnecessary . . . and of absolutely no value in diagnosis or treatment." Maurice Pappworth, "Dangerous Head That May Rule the Heart," *Perspective*, pp. 67–70.

[180]Peter Schrag, Diane Divoky. *The Myth of the Hyperactive Child. And Other Means of Child Control.* Pantheon, 1975. The definitive repertory on an "entire generation slowly being conditioned to distrust its own instincts, to regard its deviation from the narrowing standards of approved norms as sickness and to rely on the institutions of the state and on technology to define and engineer its "health." The book also provides a guide to the U.S. literature on the subject. Peter Schrag in personal communications with the author has not only shaped his view on the medicalization of society but has also been of invaluable help in editing parts of the definitive edition of *Medical Nemesis.* Minimal brain damage in children is as often as not a creation of Ritalin; it is a diagnosis determined by the treatment. See Roger D. Freeman, "Review of Medicine in Special Education: Medical-Behavioral Pseudorelationships," *Journal of Special Education 5* (winter–spring 1971): 93–99.

[181]Alexander R. Lucas and Morris Weiss, "Methylphenidate Hallucinosis," *Journal of the American Medical Association* 217 (1971): 1079–81. Ritalin is used for the control of minimal brain dysfunction in schoolchildren. The author questions the ethics of using a powerful agent with serious side-effects, some well defined and others suspected, for mass therapy of a condition that is ill-defined. See also Barbara Fish, "The One-Child–One-Drug Myth of Stimulants in Hyperkinesis," *Archives of General Psychiatry* 25 (September 1971): 193–203. Considerable permanent damage has probably been done to hyperactive children treated with ampheta-

simple and otherwise benign examinations turn into risks when multiplied. When a test is associated with several others, it has considerably greater power to harm than when it is conducted by itself. Often tests provide guidance in the choice of therapy. Unfortunately, as the tests turn more complex and are multiplied, their results frequently provide guidance only in selecting the form of intervention which the patient may survive, and not necessarily that which will help him. Worst of all, when people have lived through complex positive laboratory diagnosis, unharmed or not, they have incurred a high risk of being submitted to therapy that is odious, painful, crippling, and expensive. No wonder that physicians tend to delay longer than laymen before going to see their own doctor and that they are in worse shape when they get there.[182]

Routine performance of early diagnostic tests on large populations guarantees the medical scientist a broad base from which to select the cases that best fit existing treatment facilities or are most useful in the attainment of research goals, whether or not the therapies cure, rehabilitate, or soothe. In the process, people are strengthened in their belief that they are machines whose durability depends on visits to the maintenance shop, and are thus not only obliged but also pressured to foot the bill for the market research and the sales activities of the medical establishment.

Diagnosis always intensifies stress, defines incapacity, imposes inactivity, and focuses apprehension on nonrecovery, on uncertainty, and on one's dependence upon future medical findings, all of which amounts to a loss of autonomy for self-definition. It also isolates a person in a special role, separates him from the normal and healthy, and requires submission to the authority of specialized personnel. Once a so-

---

mines for a condition possibly due to biochemical stress from lead poisoning: D. Bryce-Smith and H. A. Waldron, "Lead, Behavior, and Criminality," *Ecologist* 4, no. 10 (1975).

[182]Barbara Blackwell, *The Literature of Delay in Seeking Medical Care for Chronic Illnesses,* Health Education Monograph no. 16 (San Francisco: Society for Public Health Education, 1963).

ciety organizes for a preventive disease-hunt, it gives epidemic proportions to diagnosis. This ultimate triumph of therapeutic culture[183] turns the independence of the average healthy person into an intolerable form of deviance.

In the long run the main activity of such an inner-directed systems society leads to the phantom production of life expectancy as a commodity. By equating statistical man with biologically unique men, an insatiable demand for finite resources is created. The individual is subordinated to the greater "needs" of the whole, preventive procedures become compulsory,[184] and the right of the patient to withhold consent to his own treatment vanishes as the doctor argues that he must submit to diagnosis, since society cannot afford the burden of curative procedures that would be even more expensive.[185]

Terminal Ceremonies

Therapy reaches its apogee in the death-dance around the terminal patient.[186] At a cost of between $500 and $2,000 per day,[187] celebrants in white and

---

[183]Philip Rieff, *Triumph of the Therapeutic: Uses of Faith after Freud* (New York: Harper Torchbook, 1968), argues that the hospital has succeeded the church and the parliament as the archetypical institution of Western culture.

[184]Like policemen in pursuit of crime prevention, doctors are now given the benefit of the doubt if they harm the patient. William A. Westley, "Violence and the Police," *American Journal of Sociology* 59 (July 1953): 34–41, found that one-third of all people in a small industrial city, asked, "When do you think a policeman is justified in roughing up a man?" said they believed it was legitimate to use violence just to coerce respect for the police.

[185]Joseph Cooper, "A Non-Physician Looks at Medical Utopia," *Journal of the American Medical Association* 197 (1966): 697–9.

[186]Orville Brim et al., eds., *The Dying Patient* (New York: Russell Sage, 1960). An anthology with a bibliography for each contribution. First deals with the spectrum of technical analysis and decision-making in which health professionals engage when they are faced with the task of determining the circumstances "under which an individual's death should occur." Provides a series of recommendations about what might be done to make this engineering process "somewhat less graceless and less distasteful for the patient, his family and, most of all, the attending personnel."

[187]Though the cost of intensive terminal care has easily doubled just in the last 4 years, it is still useful to consult Robert J. Glaser,

blue envelop what remains of the patient in antiseptic smells.[188] The more exotic the incense and the pyre, the more death mocks the priest.[189] The religious use of medical technique has come to prevail over its technical purpose, and the line separating the physician from the mortician has been blurred.[190] Beds are filled with bodies neither dead nor alive.[191] The

---

"Innovation and Heroic Acts in Prolonging Life," in Brim et al., *The Dying Patient,* chap. 6, pp. 102–28.

[188]Richard A. Kalish, "Death and Dying: A Briefly Annotated Bibliography," in Brim et al., *The Dying Patient,* pp. 327–80. An annotated bibliographic survey of English-language literature on dying, limited mainly to items which deal with contemporary professional activity, decision-making, and technology in the hospital. This is an extract from a much larger list by the same author. For complementing items see Austin H. Kutscher, Jr., and Austin H. Kutscher, *A Bibliography of Books on Death, Bereavement, Loss and Grief, 1953–68* (New York: Health Sciences Publishing Corp., 1969).

[189]Increase in medical expenditures can add no more to the average life expectancy of entire populations in rich countries, from the U.S. to China. It can add significantly only to the life-span of the very young in most of the poorer countries. This has been dealt with in the first chapter. The ability of medicine to affect the survival rates of small groups of people selected by medical diagnosis is something else. Antibiotics have enormously increased the chances of surviving pneumonia; oral rehydration, the probability of surviving dysentery or cholera. Such effective interventions are overwhelmingly of the cheap and simple kind. Their administration under the control of a professional physician may have become a cultural must for Americans, but it is not yet so for Mexicans. A third issue is the ability of medical treatment to increase the chances for survival among an even smaller proportion of people: those affected by acute conditions that can be cured thanks to speedy and complex hospital care, and those affected by degenerative conditions in which complex technology can obtain remissions. For this group the rule applies: the more expensive the treatment, the less the value in terms of added life expectancy. A fourth group are the terminally ill: money tends to prolong dying only by starting it earlier.

[190]For the language with which Americans referred to the corpse just before physicians intruded into the mortician's business, see Jessica Mitford, *The American Way of Death* (New York: Simon & Schuster, 1963).

[191]Under new names the "zombie" has become an important subject in medicolegal disputations, to judge from the inflation of literature on conflicting claims of death and life over the body. Institute of Society, Ethics, and the Life Sciences, Research Group on Ethical, Social, and Legal Issues in Genetic Counseling and Genetic Engineering, "Ethical and Social Issues in Screening for

conjuring doctor perceives himself as a manager of crisis.[192] In an insidious way he provides each citizen at the last hour with an encounter with society's deadening dream of infinite power.[193] Like any crisis manager of bank, state, or couch, he plans self-defeating strategies and commandeers resources which, in their uselessness and futility, seem all the more grotesque. At the last moment, he promises to each patient that claim on absolute priority for which most people regard themselves as too unimportant.

The ritualization of crisis, a general trait of a morbid society, does three things for the medical functionary. It provides him with a license that usually only the military can claim. Under the stress of crisis, the professional who is believed to be in command

---

Genetic Disease," *New England Journal of Medicine* 286 (1972): 1129–32. A good summary of current opinions on the criteria for determining that death has occurred. The authors carefully separate this issue from any attempt to define death. Alexandre Capron and Leon R. Kass, "A Statutory Definition of the Standards for Determining Human Death: An Appraisal and a Proposal," *University of Pennsylvania Law Review* 121 (November 1972): 87–118. An introduction to the legal aspects of the physician's intrusion into the gravedigger's domain.

[192]This spread of legitimacy for the institutional management of crisis has enormous political potential because it prepares for irreversible crisis government. Just as Weber could argue that Puritan wealth was an unintended consequence of the anxiety aroused by the doctrine of predestination, so a moralist historian of Tawney's fiber might argue that readiness for technofascism is the unintended consequence of a society that voted for terminal care to be paid for by national insurance.

[193]By "ritualization" crisis is transformed from an urgent occasion for personal integration (Erikson) into a stress situation (Robinson, for some discussion) in which a bureaucratic apparatus is forced into action in pursuit of a goal for which, by its very nature, it cannot be organized. Under such circumstances, the institution's make-believe functions will take the upper hand. This must happen when medicine pursues a "dying policy." The confusion is enhanced by the use of a word such as "dying" or "decision," which designates action that springs from intimacy in a context devoid of it. Erik Erikson, "Psychoanalysis and Ongoing History: Problems of Identity, Hatred, and Nonviolence," *American Journal of Psychiatry* 122 (September 1965): 241–53. James Robinson, *The Concept of Crisis in Decision-Making,* Symposi Studies Series no. 11 (Washington, D.C.: National Institute of Social and Behavioral Science, 1962).

can easily presume immunity from the ordinary rules of justice and decency. He who is assigned control over death ceases to be an ordinary human. As with the director of a triage, his killing is covered by policy.[194] More important, his entire performance takes place in the aura of crisis.[195] Because they form a charmed borderland not quite of this world, the time-span and the community space claimed by the medical enterprise are as sacred as their religious and military counterparts. Not only does the medicalization of terminal care ritualize macabre dreams and enlarge professional license for obscene endeavors: the escalation of terminal treatments removes from the physician all need to prove the technical effectiveness of those resources he commands.[196] There are no limits to his power to demand more and ever more. Finally, the patient's death places the physician beyond potential control and criticism. In the last glance of the patient and in the life-long perspective of the "morituri" there is no hope, but only the physician's last expectation.[197] The orientation of any institution towards "crisis" justifies enormous ordinary ineffectiveness.[198]

---

[194]Leonard Lewin, *Triage* (New York: Dial Press, 1972), raises the issue of society committed to dying policy in a novel which, unfortunately, does not compare with his previous *Report from Iron Mountain.*

[195]Valentina Borremans and Ivan Illich, "Dying Policy," manuscript prepared for *Encyclopedia of Bio-Ethics,* Kennedy Institute, Washington, D.C., 1976. The authors agreed to contribute the entry under the title proposed by the editors of the encyclopedia precisely to highlight the fact that the combination of the intransitive verb "to die" and the bureaucratic term "policy" constitutes the supreme attack on language and reason.

[196]He who successfully claims power in an emergency suspends and can destroy rational evaluation. The insistence of the physician on his exclusive capacity to evaluate and solve individual crises moves him symbolically into the neighborhood of the White House.

[197]For the author's view on the distinction between hope and expectation as two opposed future-oriented attitudes, see Ivan Illich, "The Dawn of Epithimethean Man," paper prepared for a symposium in honor of Erich Fromm. Expectation is an optimistic or pessimistic reliance on institutionalized technical means; hope, a trusting readiness to be surprised by another person.

[198]"Crisis" thus becomes the red herring used by the executive to heighten his power in inverse proportion to the services he

Hospital death is now endemic.[199] In the last twenty-five years the percentage of Americans who die in a hospital has grown by a third.[200] The percentage of hospital deaths in other countries has grown even faster. Death without medical presence becomes synonymous with romantic pigheadedness, privilege, or disaster. The cost of a citizen's last days has increased by an estimated 1,200 percent, much faster than that of over-all health-care. Simultaneously, at least in the United States, funeral costs have stabilized; their growth rate has come in line with the rise of the general consumer-price index. The most elaborate phase of the terminal ceremonies now surrounds the dying patient and has been separated, under medical control, from the removal exequies and the burial of what remains. In a switch of lavish expenditure from tomb to ward, reflecting the horror of dying without medical assistance,[201] the insured pay for participation in their own funeral rites.[202]

---

renders. It also becomes, in ever new combinations (energy crisis, authority crisis, East-West crisis), an inexhaustible subject for well-financed research by scientists paid to give to "crisis" the scholarly content that justifies the grantor. See Renzo Tomatis, *La ricerca illimitata* (Milan: Feltrinelli, 1975).

[199]The term "hospital death" is used here to designate all deaths that happen in a hospital, and not only that 10% of the total which are "associated with a diagnostic or therapeutic procedure which is considered a contributing, precipitating or primary cause of obitus." Elihu Schimmel, "The Hazards of Hospitalization," *Annals of Internal Medicine* 60 (January 1964): 100–16.

[200]Monroe Lerner, "When, Why, and Where People Die," in Brim et al., *The Dying Patient*, pp. 5–29. Gives breakdowns of this evolution between 1955 and 1967 by cause of death, color, and region of the U.S.

[201]Erwin H. Ackerknecht, "Death in the History of Medicine," *Bulletin of the History of Medicine* 42 (1968): 19–23. For the elites of the Enlightenment, death became different and far more frightening than it had been for earlier generations. Apparently death became a kind of secularized hell and a major medical concern. "Live tests" by trumpet-blowing (Professor Hufeland) and electric shock (Creve) were introduced. Bichat's *Recherches physiologiques sur la vie et la mort* (1800) ended the anti–apparent-death movement in medicine as suddenly as Lancisi's work had started it in 1707.

[202] All societies seem to have distinguished stages by which the living pass into the grave. I will deal with these in chapter 9, and show how the renewed concern with the taxonomy of decay is consistent with other contemporary regressions to primitive fascinations.

Fear of unmedicated death was first felt by eighteenth-century elites who refused religious assistance and rejected belief in the afterlife.[203] A new wave of this fear has now swept rich and poor, and has combined with egalitarian pathos to create a new category of goods: those which are "terminally" scarce, because they are commandeered by the physician in high-cost death chambers. To distribute these goods, a new branch of legal[204] and ethical literature has arisen to deal with the question how to exclude some, select others, and justify choices of life-prolonging techniques and ways of making death more comfortable and acceptable.[205] Taken as a whole, this literature tells a remarkable story about the mind of the contemporary jurist and philosopher. Most of the authors do not even ask whether the techniques that sustain their speculations have in fact proved to be life-prolonging. Naïvely, they go along with the delusion that ongoing rituals that are costly must be useful. In this way law and ethics bolster belief in the value of policies that regulate politically innocuous medical equality at the point of death.

The modern fear of unhygienic death makes life appear like a race towards a terminal scramble and has broken personal self-confidence in a unique

---

[203]Margot Augener, "Scheintod als medizinisches Problem im 18. Jahrhundert," *Mitteilungen zur Geschichte der Medizin und der Naturwissenschaften*, nos. 6–7 (1967). The secularized fear of hell on the part of the enlightened rich focused on the horror of being buried alive. It also led to the creation of philanthropic foundations dedicated to the succor of the drowning or the burning.

[204]"Scarce Medical Resources," editorial, *Columbia Law Review* 69 (April 1969): 690–2. A review article based on interviews with several dozen U.S. experts. Describes and evaluates the current policies of exclusion and selection from a legal point of view. Uncritically accepts the probable effectiveness of the techniques supposed to be in extreme demand.

[205]Sharmon Sollito and Robert M. Veatch, *Bibliography of Society, Ethics and the Life Sciences*, a Hastings Center Publication (Hastings-on-Hudson, N.Y., 1974). J. R. Elkinton, "The Literature of Ethical Problems in Medicine," pts. 1, 2, 3, *Annals of Internal Medicine* 73 (September 1970): 495–8; (October 1970): 662–6; (November 1970): 863–70. These are mutually complementary introductions to the ethical literature.

way.[206] It has fostered the belief that man today has lost the autonomy to recognize when his time has come and to take his death into his own hands.[207] The doctor's refusal to recognize the point at which he has ceased to be useful as a healer[208] and to withdraw when death shows on his patient's face[209] has made him into an agent of evasion or outright dissimulation.[210] The patient's unwillingness to die on his own makes him pathetically dependent. He has now lost his faith in his ability to die, the terminal shape

---

[206] Hermann Feifel, "Physicians Consider Death," in *Proceedings of the American Psychological Association Convention* (Washington, D.C.: the Association, 1967), pp. 201–2. Physicians seem significantly more afraid of death than either the physically sick or the normal healthy individual. The argument could lead to the thesis that physicians are now carriers of infectious fright.

[207] *Euthanasia: An Annotated Bibliography,* Euthanasia Educational Fund, 250 West 57th Street, New York, N.Y. 10019.

[208] The right to heal as an intransitive activity that must be exercised by the patient can enter into conflict with the assertion of the physician's right to heal, a transitive activity. For the origins of a medical right to heal, which would correspond to a professional duty, see Ludwig Edelstein, "The Professional Ethics of the Greek Physician," *Bulletin of the History of Medicine* 30 (September–October 1956): 391–419. Walter Reich raises the contemporary issue about the substance in the physician-patient contract when the disease turns from curable to terminal and therefore a "healer contract" comes to an end. Walter Reich, "The Physician's 'Duty' to Preserve Life," *Hastings Center Report* 5 (April 1975): 14–15.

[209] The recognition of the *facies hippocratica,* the signs of approaching death that indicated to the physician the point at which curative efforts had to be abandoned, was part of the medical curricula until the end of the 19th century. On this subject, see chapter 8.

[210] Fred Davis, "Uncertainty in Medical Prognosis, Clinical and Functional," *American Journal of Sociology* 66 (July 1960): 41–7. Davis examines the doctor's behavior when an unfavorable prognosis of impairment or death becomes certain, and finds widespread cultivation of uncertainty by dissimulation or evasion. Dissimulation feeds Dr. Slop or Dr. Knock, who proffers clinically unsubstantiated diagnoses to curry favorable opinion by selling unwarranted placebos. Evasion, or the failure to communicate a clinically substantiated prognosis, keeps the patient and his family in the dark, lets them find out "in a natural sort of way," allows the doctor to avoid loss of his time—and scenes, and permits the doctor to pursue treatments the patient would have rejected had he known they cannot cure. Uncertainty is often cultivated as a conspiracy between doctor and patient to avoid acceptance of the irreversible, a category which does not fit their ethos.

that health can take, and has made the right to be professionally killed into a major issue.[211]

Several unexamined expectations are interwoven in the cultural orientation towards death in the wards. People think that hospitalization will reduce their pain or that they will probably live longer in the hospital. Neither is likely to be true. Of those admitted with a fatal condition to the average British clinic, 10 percent died on the day of arrival, 30 percent within a week, 75 percent within a month, and 97 percent within three months.[212] In homes for terminal care, 56 percent were dead within a week of admission. In terminal cancer, there is no difference in life expectancy between those who end in the home and those who die in the hospital. Only a quarter of terminal cancer patients need special nursing at home, and then only during their last weeks. For more than half, suffering will be limited to feeling feeble and uncomfortable, and what pain there is can usually be relieved.[213] But by staying at home, they avoid the exile, loneliness, and indignities which, in

---

[211]Sissela Bok et al., "The Dilemmas of Euthanasia," *Bioscience* 23 (August 1973): 461–78. It is often overlooked that euthanasia, or the medical termination of human life, could not have been an important issue before terminal care was medicalized. At present, most legal and ethical literature dealing with the legitimacy and the moral status of such professional contributions to the acceleration of death is of very limited value, because it does not call in question the legal and ethical status of medicalization, which created the issue in the first place. H. L. Hart, *Law, Liberty and Morality* (Stanford, Calif.: Stanford Univ. Press, 1963). By arguing that the law ought to take a neutral position, Hart goes perhaps furthest in this discussion. On one side the travesty of ethics takes the form of forced sale of medical products at literally any cost. Freeman states that "the death of an unoperated patient is an unacceptable means of alleviating sufferings" not only for the patient but also for his family: John M. Freeman, "Whose Suffering?" and Robert E. Cooke, "Is There a Right to Die—Quickly?" *Journal of Pediatrics* 80 (May 1972): 904–8. On the other hand, even the spokesmen in favor of terminal self-medication with pain-killers proceed on the assumption that in this as in any other consumption of drugs, the patient must buy what another selects for him.

[212]John Hinton, *Dying* (Baltimore: Penguin Books, 1974).

[213]Institute of Medicine of Chicago, *Terminal Care for Cancer Patients* (Chicago: Central Service for the Chronically Ill, 1950).

all but exceptional hospitals, awaits them.[214] Poor blacks seem to know this and upset the hospital routine by taking their dying home. Opiates are not available on demand. Patients who have severe pains over months or years, which narcotics could make tolerable, are as likely to be refused medication in the hospital as at home, lest they form a habit in their incurable but not directly fatal condition.[215] Finally, people believe that hospitalization increases their chances of surviving a crisis. With some clear-cut exceptions, on this point too, more often than not, they are wrong. More people die now because crisis intervention is hospital-centered than can be saved through the superior techniques the hospital can provide. In the poor countries many more children have died of cholera or diarrhea during the last ten years because they were not rehydrated on time with a simple solution forced down their throats: care was centered on sophisticated intravenous rehydration at a distant hospital.[216] In rich countries the deaths caused by the use of evacuation equipment are beginning to balance the number of lives thus saved. Hospital "worship" is unrelated to the hospital's performance.

Like any other growth industry, the health system directs its products where demand seems unlimited: into defense against death. An increasing percentage of newly acquired tax funds is allocated towards life-extension technology for terminal patients. Complex bureaucracies sanctimoniously select for dialysis maintenance one in six or one in three of those Americans who are threatened by kidney failure. The patient-elect is conditioned to desire the

---

[214]David Sudnow, *Passing On: The Social Organization of Dying* (Englewood Cliffs, N.J.: Prentice-Hall, 1967). Described in its introduction as "salutary reading for the laymen whose contact with the terminal phase of human life is limited to occasional encounters," this book should cure one of any desire for professional assistance.

[215]Exton-Smith, "Terminal Illness in the Aged."

[216]For a summary of several studies, see International Bank for Reconstruction and Development, *Health Sector Policy Paper* (Washington, D.C., March 1975), p. 34.

scarce privilege of dying in exquisite torture.[217] As a doctor observes in an account of the treatment of his own illness, much time and effort must go into preventing suicide during the first and sometimes the second year that the artificial kidney may add to life.[218] In a society where the majority die under the control of public authority, the solemnities formerly surrounding legalized homicide or execution adorn the terminal ward. The sumptuous treatment of the comatose takes the place of the doomed man's breakfast in other cultures.[219]

Public fascination with high-technology care and death can be understood as a deep-seated need for the engineering of miracles. Intensive care is but the culmination of a public worship organized around a medical priesthood struggling against death.[220]

---

[217]"Improvements in artificial kidneys are needed, as borne out by the fact that uremic patients often are subjectively worse for a period after dialysis even though their blood chemistry is apparently near normal. Possible explanations are the nonremoval of an unknown 'uremic factor' or more likely the unwanted removal of a needed factor from the blood, or perhaps some subtle injury to the blood by the kidney machine." Rushmer, *Medical Engineering*, p. 314.

[218]C. H. Calland, "Iatrogenic Problems in End-Stage Renal Failure," *New England Journal of Medicine* 287 (1972): 334–8. An autobiographical account of a medical doctor in such terminal treatment.

[219]Hans von Hentig, *Vom Ursprung der Henkersmahlzeit* (Tübingen: Mohr, 1958). The medicalization of death has enormously increased the percentage of people whose death happens under bureaucratic control. In his encyclopedic study of the breakfast offered a condemned man by his executioner, Hentig concludes that there exists a deep-felt need to lavish favors on persons who die in a publicly determined way. Usually this favor takes the form of a sumptuous meal. Even during World War I soldiers still exchange cigarettes, and the firing-squad commander offered a last cigarette. Terminal treatment in war, prison, and hospital has now been depersonalized. Intensive care for the dying can also be seen as a funeral gift for the unburied.

[220]Stephen P. Strickland, *Politics, Science and Dread Disease: A Short History of the United States Medical Research Policy*, Commonwealth Fund Series (Cambridge: Harvard Univ. Press, 1972). Strickland describes how the U.S. government medical research policy got under way with the 1927 proposal by a senator to post a $5 million reward for the person who collared the worst killer, namely cancer. Gives the history of the boom in cancer

The willingness of the public to finance these activities expresses a desire for the nontechnical functions of medicine. Cardiac intensive-care units, for example, have high visibility and no proven statistical gain for the care of the sick. They require three times the equipment and five times the staff needed for normal patient care; 12 percent of all graduate hospital nurses in the United States work in this heroic medicine. This gaudy enterprise is supported, like a liturgy of old, by the extortion of taxes, by the solicitation of gifts, and by the procurement of victims. Large-scale random samples have been used to compare the mortality and recovery rates of patients served by these units with those of patients given home treatment. So far they have demonstrated no advantage. The patients who have suffered cardiac infarction themselves tend to express a preference for home care; they are frightened by the hospital, and in a crisis would rather be close to people they know. Careful statistical findings have confirmed their intuition: the higher mortality of those benefitted by mechanical care in the hospital is usually ascribed to fright.[221]

Black Magic

Technical intervention in the physical and biochemical make-up of the patient or of his environment is not, and never has been, the sole function of medical institutions.[222] The removal of pathogens

---

research. The U.S. government now spends more than $500 million per year on it.

[221]H. G. Mather et al., "Acute Myocardial Infarction: Home and Hospital Treatment," *British Medical Journal,* 1971, 3:334–8.

[222]John Powles has made this argument; see "On the Limitations of Modern Medicine," in *Science, Medicine and Man* (London: Pergamon, 1973), 1:1–30. An increasingly large proportion of the contemporary disease burden is man-made; engineering intervention in sickness is not making much progress as a strategy. The continued insistence on this strategy can be explained only if it serves nontechnical purposes. Diminishing returns within medicine are a specific instance of a wider crisis in industrial man's relationship to his environment. J. P. Dupuy, S. Karsenty, La logique cachée de la croissance de l'institution médicale. in:/sans indication de la pub-

and the application of remedies (effective or not) are by no means the sole way of mediating between man and his disease. Even in those circumstances in which the physician is technically equipped to play the technical role to which he aspires, he inevitably also fulfills religious, magical, ethical, and political functions. In each of these functions the contemporary physician is more pathogen than healer or just anodyne.

Magic or healing through ceremonies is clearly one of the important traditional functions of medicine.[223] In magic the healer manipulates the setting and the stage. In a somewhat impersonal way he establishes an ad hoc relationship between himself and a group of individuals. Magic works if and when the intent of patient and magician coincides,[224] though it took scientific medicine considerable time to recognize its own practitioners as part-time magicians. To distinguish the doctor's professional exercise of white magic from his function as engineer (and to spare him the charge of being a quack), the term "placebo" was created. Whenever a sugar pill works because it is given by the doctor, the sugar pill acts as a placebo. A placebo (Latin for "I will please") pleases not only the patient but the administering physician as well.[225]

In high cultures, religious medicine is something quite distinct from magic.[226] The major religions

---

lication/no. 3, été 1975. pp. 179–202. Describes the economic mechanisms by which the health-care system has been turned primarily into an enterprise for the production and consumption of symbols.

[223]M. Bartels, *Die Medizin der Naturvölker* (Leipzig: Grieben, 1893). A classic on the magical element in the medicine of primitive peoples.

[224]William J. Goode, "Religion and Magic," in Goode, ed., *Religion Among the Primitives* (New York: Free Press, 1951), pp. 50–4.

[225]On the history of medical studies of the placebo effect and the evolution of the term, see Arthur K. Shapiro, "A Contribution to a History of the Placebo Effect," *Behavioral Science* 5 (April 1960): 109–35.

[226]The distinction between the magical elimination, religious interpretation, or ethical socialization of suffering and its technical manipulation and legal control deserves much more detailed analysis. I introduce these distinctions only to clarify that (1) medical technique does have nontechnical effects (2) some of which cannot

reinforce resignation to misfortune and offer a rationale, a style, and a community setting in which suffering can become a dignified performance. The opportunities offered by the acceptance of suffering can be differently explained in each of the great traditions: as karma accumulated through past incarnations; as an invitation to Islam, the surrender to God; or as an opportunity for closer association with the Savior on the Cross. High religion stimulates personal responsibility for healing, sends ministers for sometimes pompous and sometimes effective consolation, provides saints as models, and usually provides a framework for the practice of folk medicine. In our kind of secular society religious organizations are left with only a small part of their former ritual healing roles. One devout Catholic might derive intimate strength from personal prayer, some marginal groups of recent arrivals in São Paolo might routinely heal their ulcers in Afro-Latin dance cults, and Indians in the valley of the Ganges still seek health in the singing of the Vedas. But such things have only a remote parallel in societies beyond a certain per capita GNP. In these industrialized societies secular institutions run the major myth-making ceremonies.[227]

The separate cults of education, transportation, and mass communication promote, under different names, the same social myth which Voeglin[228] describes as contemporary gnosis. Common to a gnostic world-view and its cult are six characteristics: (1) it is practiced by members of a movement who are dis-

---

be considered economic or social externalities (3) because they specifically influence health levels. (4) These health-related latent functions do have a complex, multilayered structure and (5) more often than not spoil health.

[227]By myths I here mean set behavior patterns which have the ability to generate among the participants a blindness to or tolerance for the divergence between the rationalization reinforced by the celebration of the ritual and the social consequences produced by this same celebration, which are in direct contradiction to the myth. For an analysis see Max Gluckman, *Order and Rebellion in Tribal Africa* (New York: Free Press, 1963).

[228]Eric Voeglin, *Science, Politics and Gnosticism,* trans. William Fitzpatrick (Chicago: Regnery, 1968).

satisfied with the world as it is because they see it as intrinsically poorly organized. Its adherents are (2) convinced that salvation from this world is possible (3) at least for the elect and (4) can be brought about within the present generation. Gnostics further believe that this salvation depends (5) on technical actions which are reserved (6) to initiates who monopolize the special formula for it. All these religious beliefs underlie the social organization of technological medicine, which in turn ritualizes and celebrates the nineteenth-century ideal of progress.

Among the important nontechnical functions of medicine, a third one is ethical rather than magical, secular rather than religious. It does not depend on a conspiracy into which the sorcerer enters with his adept, nor on myths to which the priest gives form, but on the shape which medical culture gives to interpersonal relations. Medicine can be so organized that it motivates the community to deal in a more or less personal fashion with the frail, the decrepit, the tender, the crippled, the depressed, and the manic. By fostering a certain type of social character, a society's medicine could effectively lessen the suffering of the diseased by assigning an active role to all members of the community in the compassionate tolerance for and the selfless assistance of the weak.[229] Medicine could regulate society's gift relationships.[230] Cultures where compassion for the unfortunate, hospitality for the crippled, leeway for the troubled, and respect for the old have been developed can, to a large extent, integrate the majority of their members into everyday life.

---

[229]The social ordering of compassion, nurture, and celebration has been the most effective aspect of primitive medicine; see Erwin H. Ackerknecht, "Natural Diseases and Rational Treatment in Primitive Medicine," *Bulletin of the History of Medicine* 19 (May 1946): 467–97.

[230]Richard M. Titmuss, *The Gift Relationship* (New York: Pantheon, 1971), compares the market for human blood under U.S. commercial and British socialized medical systems, shows the immense superiority of British blood transfusions, and argues that the greater effectiveness of the British approach is due to the lower level of commercialization.

Healers can be priests of the gods, lawgivers, magicians, mediums, barber-pharmacists, or scientific advisers.[231] No common name with even the approximate semantic range covered by our "doctor" existed in Europe before the fourteenth century.[232] In Greece the repairman, used mostly for slaves, was respected early, though he was not on a level with the healing philospher or even with the gymnast for the free.[233] Republican Rome considered the specialized curers a disreputable lot. Laws on water supply, drainage, garbage removal, and military training, combined with the state cult of healing gods, were considered sufficient; grandmother's brew and the army sanitarian were not dignified by special attention. Until Julius Caesar gave citizenship to the first group of Asclepiads in 46 B.C., this privilege was refused to Greek physicians and healing priests.[234] The Arabs honored the physician;[235] the Jews left health care to the quality of the ghetto or, with a bad conscience, brought in the Arab physician.[236] Medicine's several functions combined in different ways in different roles. The first occupation to monopolize health care

---

[231]Only in Chaucer's time did a common name for all healers appear: Vern L. Bullough, "Medical Study at Medieval Oxford," *Speculum* 36 (1961): 600–12.

[232]"The Term 'Doctor,'" *Journal of the History of Medicine and Allied Sciences* 18 (1963): 284–7.

[233]Louis Cohn-Haft, *The Public Physician of Ancient Greece* (Northampton, Mass.: Smith College, 1956).

[234]Adalberto Pazzini, *Storia della medicina,* 2 vols. (Milan: Società editrice libraria, 1947).

[235]For Arab medicine in general, consult Lucien Leclerc, *Histoire de la médecine arabe: Exposé complet des traductions du grec: Les Sciences en Orient, leur transmission à l'Occident par les traductions latines,* 2 vols. (1876; reprint ed., New York: Franklin, 1971); Manfred Ullmann, *Die Medizin im Islam* (Leiden: Brill, 1970), an exhaustive guide. But see also the judgment of Ibn Khaldun, *The Muqaddimah: An Introduction to History,* trans. Franz Rosenthal, Bollingen Series XLIII, 3 vols. (Princeton, N.J.: Princeton Univ. Press, 1967). For a critical review of Arabic contributions to the Western image of the doctor, see Heinrich Schipperges, "Ideologie und Historiographie des Arabismus," *Sudhoffs Archiv,* suppl. 1, 1961.

[236]Jacob Marcus, *Communal Sick-Care in the German Ghetto* (Cincinnati: Hebrew Union College Press, 1947). This book provides reasons for bad conscience for relying on outsiders.

is that of the physician of the late twentieth century.

Paradoxically, the more attention is focused on the technical mastery of disease, the larger becomes the symbolic and nontechnical function performed by medical technology. The less proof there is that more money increases survival rates in a given branch of cancer treatment, the more money will go to the medical divisions deployed in that special theater of operations. Only goals unrelated to treatment, such as jobs for the specialists, equal access by the poor, symbolic consolation for patients, or experimentation on humans, can explain the expansion of lung-cancer surgeries during the last twenty-five years. Not only white coats, masks, antiseptics, and ambulance sirens but entire branches of medicine continue to be financed because they have been invested with nontechnical, usually symbolic power.

Willy-nilly the modern doctor is thus forced into symbolic, nontechnical roles. Nontechnical functions prevail in the removal of adenoids: more than 90 percent of all tonsillectomies performed in the United States are technically unnecessary, yet 20 to 30 percent of all children still undergo the operation. One in a thousand dies directly as a consequence of the operation and 16 in a thousand suffer from serious complications. All lose valuable immunity mechanisms. All are subjected to emotional aggression: they are incarcerated in a hospital, separated from their parents, and introduced to the unjustified and more often than not pompous cruelty of the medical establishment.[237] The child learns to be exposed to technicians who, in his presence, use a foreign language in which they make judgments about his body; he learns that his body may be invaded by strangers for reasons they alone know; and he is made to feel proud to live in a country where social security pays for such a medical initiation into the reality of life.[238]

---

[237] S. D. Lipton, "On Psychology of Childhood Tonsillectomy," in R. S. Eissler et al., eds., *Psychoanalytic Study of the Child* (New York: International Univs. Press, 1962), 17:363–417; reprinted in Anthologia A8 (Cuernavaca: CIDOC, 1974).

[238] Julius A. Roth, "Ritual and Magic in the Control of Con-

Physical participation in a ritual is not a necessary condition for initiation into the myth which the ritual is organized to generate. Medical spectator sports cast powerful spells. I happened to be in Rio de Janeiro and in Lima when Dr. Christiaan Barnard was touring there. In both cities he was able to fill the major football stadium twice in one day with crowds who hysterically acclaimed his macabre ability to replace human hearts. Medical-miracle treatments of this kind have worldwide impact. Their alienating effect reaches people who have no access to a neighborhood clinic, much less to a hospital. It provides them with an abstract assurance that salvation through science is possible. The experience in the stadium at Rio prepared me for the evidence I was shown shortly afterwards which proved that the Brazilian police have so far been the first to use life-extending equipment in the torture of prisoners. Such extreme abuse of medical techniques seems grotesquely coherent with the dominant ideology of medicine.

The unintended nontechnical influence that medical technique exercises on society's health can, of course, be positive.[239] An unnecessary shot of penicillin can magically restore confidence and appetite.[240] A contraindicated operation can solve a marriage problem and reduce symptoms of disease in both partners.[241] Not only the doctor's sugar pills but even

---

tagion," *American Sociological Review* 22 (June 1957): 310–14. Describes how doctors come to believe in magic. Belief in the danger of contagion from tuberculosis patients leads to ritualized procedures and irrational practices. For instance, the rules compelling patients to wear protective masks are strictly enforced when they go to X-ray services but not when they go to movies or socials.

239Arthur K. Shapiro, "Factors Contributing to the Placebo Effect: Their Implications for Psychotherapy," *American Journal of Psychotherapy* 18, suppl. 1 (March 1964): 73–88.

240Otto Lippross, *Logik und Magie in der Medizin* (Munich: Lehmann, 1969), pp. 198–218. Lippross argues, and documents his belief, that most effective *healing* depends on the physician's choice of the method that most suits his personality. For bibliography, see pp. 196–218.

241Henry K. Beecher, "Surgery as Placebo: A Quantitative Study of Bias," *Journal of the American Medical Association* 176 (1961):

his poisons can be powerful placebos. But this is not the prevailing result of the nontechnical side-effects of medical technology. It can be argued that in precisely those narrow areas in which high-cost medicine has become more specifically effective, its symbolic side-effects have become overwhelmingly health-denying:[242] the traditional white medical magic that supported the patient's own efforts to heal has turned black.[243]

To a large extent, social iatrogenesis can be explained as a negative placebo, as a *nocebo* effect.[244] Overwhelmingly the nontechnical side-effects of biomedical interventions do powerful damage to health. The intensity of the black-magic influence of a medical procedure does not depend on its being technically effective. The effect of the nocebo, like that of the placebo, is largely independent of what the physician does.

Medical procedures turn into *black magic* when, instead of mobilizing his self-healing powers, they transform the sick man into a limp and mystified voyeur of his own treatment. Medical procedures turn into *sick religion* when they are performed as rituals that focus the entire expectation of the sick on science

---

1102–7. It has been long known that surgery can have placebo effects on the patient. I argue here that similar effects can be sociopolitically transmitted by highly visible interventions.

[242]Gerhard Kienle, *Arzneimittelsicherheit und Gesellschaft: Eine kritische Untersuchung* (Stuttgart: Schattauer, 1974), makes this point but deals only with the pharmacology-related sector of medical technology.

[243]Henry K. Beecher, "Nonspecific Forces Surrounding Disease and the Treatment of Disease," *Journal of the American Medical Association* 179 (1962): 437–40. "Any fear can kill, but fearful diagnosis can almost guarantee death from diagnosis." Walter B. Cannon, "Voodoo Death," *American Anthropologist* 44 (April–June 1942): 169–81. Victims of Haitian magic have ominous and persistent fears, which cause intense action of the sympatico-adrenal system and a sudden fall of blood pressure resulting in death.

[244]R. C. Pogge, "The Toxic Placebo," *Medical Times* 91 (August 1963): 778–81. S. Wolf, "Effects of Suggestion and Conditioning on the Action of Chemical Agents in Human Subjects: The Pharmacology of Placebos," *Journal of Clinical Investigation* 29 (January 1950): 100–9. G. Herzshaft, "L'Effet nocebo," *Encéphale* 58 (November–December 1969): 486–503.

and its functionaries instead of encouraging them to seek a poetic interpretation of their predicament or find an admirable example in some person—long dead or next door—who learned to suffer. Medical procedures multiply disease by *moral degradation* when they isolate the sick in a professional environment rather than providing society with the motives and disciplines that increase social tolerance for the troubled. Magical havoc, religious injury, and moral degradation generated under the pretext of a biomedical pursuit are all crucial mechanisms contributing to social iatrogenesis. They are amalgamated by the medicalization of death.

When doctors first set up shop outside the temples in Greece, India, and China, they ceased to be medicine men. When they claimed rational power over sickness, society lost the sense of the complex personage and his integrated healing which the sorcerer-shaman or curer had provided.[245] The great traditions of medical healing had left the miracle cure to priests and kings. The caste that had an "in" with the gods could call for their intervention. To the hand that wielded the sword was attributed the power to subdue not only the enemy but also the spirit. Up to the eighteenth century the king of England laid his hands every year upon those afflicted with facial tuberculosis whom physicians knew they were unable to cure.[246] Epileptics, whose ills resisted even His Majesty's touch, took refuge in the healing strength that flowed from the hands of the executioner.[247]

---

[245]Erwin Ackerknecht, "Problems of Primitive Medicine," in William A. Lessa and Evon Z. Vogt, *Reader in Comparative Religion* (New York: Harper & Row, 1965), chap. 8, pp. 394–402. Ackerknecht offers an important corrective to the Parsonian prejudice that all societies incorporate a specific kind of power in the healer. He shows that medicine man and modern physician are antagonists rather than colleagues: both take care of disease, but in all other ways they are different.

[246]Marc Bloch, *The Royal Touch: Sacred Monarchy and Scrofula in England and France,* trans. J. E. Anderson (Montreal: McGill-Queens Univ. Press, 1973).

[247]Werner Danckert, *Unehrliche Leute: Die verfemten Berufe* (Bern: Francke, 1963). Deals with the healing powers traditionally

With the rise of medical civilization and healing guilds, the physicians distinguished themselves from the quacks and the priests because they knew the limits of their art. Today the medical establishment is about to reclaim the right to perform miracles. Medicine claims the patient even when the etiology is uncertain, the prognosis unfavorable, and the therapy of an experimental nature. Under these circumstances the attempt at a "medical miracle" can be a hedge against failure, since miracles may only be hoped for and cannot, by definition, be expected. The radical monopoly over health care that the contemporary physician claims now forces him to reassume priestly and royal functions that his ancestors gave up when they became specialized as technical healers.

The medicalization of the miracle provides further insight into the social function of terminal care. The patient is strapped down and controlled like a spaceman and then displayed on television. These heroic performances serve as a rain-dance for millions, a liturgy in which realistic hopes for autonomous life are transmuted into the delusion that doctors will deliver health from outer space.

Patient Majorities

Whenever medicine's diagnostic power multiplies the sick in excessive numbers, medical professionals turn over the surplus to the management of nonmedical trades and occupations. By dumping, the medical lords divest themselves of the nuisance of low-prestige care and invest policemen, teachers, or personnel officers with a derivative medical fiefdom. Medicine retains unchecked autonomy in defining what constitutes sickness, but drops on others the task of ferreting out the sick and providing for their treatment. Only medicine knows what constitutes addiction, though policemen are supposed to

---

attributed to outcastes and marginals such as executioners, gravediggers, prostitutes, and millers. Wolfgang Dau, Schafrichter und Henker als Medici und Chirurgi. in: Materia Medica. Nordmark. 15. 1963. pp. 338–350.

know how it should be controlled. Only medicine can define brain damage, but it allows teachers to stigmatize and manage the healthy-looking cripples. When the need for a retrenchment of medical goals is discussed in medical literature, it now usually takes the shape of planned patient-dumping. Why should not the newborn and the dying, the ethnocentric, the sexually inadequate, and the neurotic, plus any number of other uninteresting and time-consuming victims of diagnostic fervor, be pushed beyond the frontiers of medicine and be transformed into clients of nonmedical therapeutic purveyors: social workers, television programmers, psychologists, personnel officers, and sex counselors?[248] This multiplication of enabling jobs that hold reflected medical prestige has created an entirely new setting for the role of the sick.

Any society, to be stable, needs certified deviance. People who look strange or who behave oddly are subversive until their common traits have been formally named and their startling behavior slotted into a recognized pigeonhole. By being assigned a name and a role, eerie, upsetting freaks are tamed, becoming predictable exceptions who can be pampered, avoided, repressed, or expelled. In most societies there are some people who assign roles to the uncommon ones; according to the prevalent social prescription, they are usually those who hold special knowledge about the nature of deviance:[249] they decide whether the deviant is possessed by a ghost, ridden by a god, infected by poison, being punished for his sin, or the victim of vengeance wrought by a witch. The agent who does this labeling does not necessarily have to be comparable to medical author-

---

[248]Dominique Wolton, *Le Nouvel Ordre sexual* (Paris: Seuil, 1974), describes the outcome of the French sexual revolution: a new "sexocracy" made up of physicians, militants, educators, and pharmacists has secularized and schooled French sexuality and "by subjecting body awareness to orthopedic management has reproduced the welfare receiver even in this intimate domain."

[249]Henry E. Sigerist, *Civilization and Disease* (Chicago: Univ. of Chicago Press, 1970).

ity: he may hold juridical, religious, or military power. By naming the spirit that underlies deviance, authority places the deviant under the control of language and custom and turns him from a threat into a support of the social system. Etiology is socially self-fulfilling: if the sacred disease is believed to be caused by divine possession, then the god speaks in the epileptic fit.[250]

Each civilization defines its own diseases.[251] What is sickness in one might be chromosomal abnormality, crime, holiness, or sin in another. Each culture creates its response to disease. For the same symptom of compulsive stealing one might be executed, treated to death, exiled, hospitalized, or given alms or tax money. Here thieves are forced to wear special clothes; there, to do penance; elsewhere, to lose a finger, or again, to be conditioned by magic or by electric shock. To postulate for every society a specifically "sick" kind of deviance with even minimal common characteristics[252] is a hazardous undertaking. The contemporary assignation of sick-roles is of a unique kind. It developed not much more than a generation before Henderson and Parsons analyzed it.[253] It defines deviance as the special legitimate

---

[250]For complementary references, refer to notes 15–18, pp. 36–7 above.

[251]T. F. Troels-Lund, *Gesundheit und Krankheit in der Anschauung alter Zeiten* (Leipzig, 1901), is an early study of the shifting frontiers of sickness in different cultures. Walther Riese, *The Conception of Disease: Its History, Its Versions and Its Nature* (New York: Philosophical Library, 1953), attempts a philosophical epistemology. For orientation on the evolution of recent discussion see David Mechanic, *Medical Sociology: A Selective View* (New York: Free Press, 1968), especially pp. 33ff.

[252]As just one example of a society without the Aesculapian role see Charles O. Frake, "The Diagnosis of Disease Among the Subanun of Mindanao," *American Anthropologist* 63 (1961): 113–32. In the sphere of making decisions about disease, differences in individual skill and knowledge receive recognition, but there is no formal status of diagnostician or even, by Subanun conception, of curer.

[253]Lawrence J. Henderson, "Physician and Patient as a Social System," *New England Journal of Medicine* 212 (1935): 819–23, was perhaps the first to suggest that the physician exonerates the sick from moral accountability for their illness. For the classical formulation of the modern, almost morality-free sick-role, see Talcott Parsons, "Illness and the Role of the Physician" (orig. 1948),

behavior of officially selected consumers within an industrial milieu.[254] Even if there were something to say for the thesis that in all societies some people are, so to speak, temporarily put out of service and pampered while being repaired, the context within which this exemption operates elsewhere cannot be compared to that of the welfare state. When he *assigns* sick-status to a client, the contemporary physician might indeed be acting in some ways similar to the sorcerer or the elder; but in belonging also to a scientific profession that *invents* the categories it assigns when consulting, the modern physician is totally unlike the healer. Medicine men engaged in the occupation of curing and exercised the art of distinguishing evil spirits from each other. They were not professionals and had no power to invent new devils. Enabling professions in their annual assemblies create the sick-roles they assign.

The roles available for an individual have always been of two kinds: those which are standardized by cultural tradition and those which are the result of bureaucratic organization. Innovation at all times meant a relative increase of the latter, rationally created roles. No doubt, engineered roles could be recovered by cultural tradition. No doubt a neat distinction between the two kinds of roles is difficult to make. But on the whole, the sick-role tended until recently to be of the traditional kind.[255] In the last

---

in Clyde Kluckhohn and Henry Murray, eds., *Personality in Nature, Society and Culture,* rev. ed. (New York: Knopf, 1953).

[254]David Robinson, *The Process of Becoming Ill* (London: Routledge, 1971), discovers a fundamental weakness in most studies done so far on the sick-role: they are based on people who finally did become patients, and deal with the person who feels ill but does not see the doctor as somebody who *delays.* He rejects the notion that illness starts with the presentation of symptoms to a professional. Most people are not patients most of the time they feel ill. Robinson studies empirically the sick behavior of nonpatients.

[255]The distinction between the *intransitive healing* by the patient and the *transitive healing* provided for him must be further refined. The latter, a service to the patient, can be provided in two profoundly distinct ways. It can be the output of an institution and its functionaries executing policies, or it can be the result of personal, spontaneous interaction within a cultural setting. The distinction has

century, however, what Foucault has called the new clinical vision has changed the proportions. The physician has increasingly abandoned his role as moralist and assumed that of enlightened scientific entrepreneur. To exonerate the sick from accountability for their illness has become a predominant task, and new scientific categories of disease have been shaped for the purpose. Medical school and clinic provide the doctor with the atmosphere in which disease, in his eyes, may become a task for biological or social technique; his patients still carry their religious and cosmic interpretations into the ward, much as the laymen once carried their secular concerns into church for Sunday service.[256] But the sick-role described by Parsons fits modern society only as long as doctors act as if treatment were usually effective and while the general public is willing to share their rosy view.[257] The mid-twentieth-century sick-role has become inadequate for describing what happens in a medical system that claims authority over people who are not yet ill, people who cannot reasonably expect to get well, and those for whom doctors have no more effective treatment than that which could be offered by their uncles or aunts. Expert selection of a few for institutional pampering was a way to use medi-

---

been elaborated by Jacques Ellul, *The Technological Society* (New York: Random House, 1964). Ellul's concept of "institutionalized values" has been subjected to the analysis of a symposium: *Katallagete* [Be Reconciled]: *Journal of the Committe of Southern Churchmen* 2 (winter–spring 1970): 1–65. The phenomenology of *personal care* has been developed by Milton Mayeroff, *On Caring* (New York: Harper & Row, 1971).

[256]Renée Fox, *Experiment Perilous: Physicians and Patients Facing the Unknown* (Glencoe, Ill.: Free Press, 1959), studies terminal patients who have consented to be used as subjects for medical experiment. Notwithstanding the prevailing logical and rational explanations for their sickness, they too grapple with it in religious, cosmic, and especially moral terms.

[257]Sickness becomes associated with high living standards and high expectations. In the first six months of 1970, 5 million working days were lost in Britain owing to industrial disputes. This has been exceeded in only 2 years since the general strike in 1926. In comparison, over 300 million working days were lost through absence due to certified sickness. Office of Health Economics, *Off Sick* (London, 1971).

cine for the purpose of stabilizing an industrial society:[258] it entailed the easily regulated entitlement of the abnormal to abnormal levels of public funds. Kept within limits, during the early twentieth century the pampering of deviants "strengthened" the cohesion of industrial society. But after a critical point social control exercised through the diagnosis of unlimited needs destroyed its own base.[259] Until proved healthy, the citizen is now presumed to be sick.[260] In a triumphantly therapeutic society, everybody can make himself into a therapist and someone else into his client.

---

[258]Clarence Karier, "Testing for Order and Control in the Corporate Liberal State," *Educational Theory* 22 (spring 1972), shows the role the Carnegie Foundation played in developing educational testing materials that can be used for social control in situations where the ability of schools to perform this task has broken down. According to Karier, tests given outside the schools are a more powerful device for discrimination than tests given within a pedagogical situation. In the same way, it can be argued that medical testing becomes an increasingly powerful means for classification and discrimination, as the number of test results accumulate for which no significant treatment is feasible. Once the patient role becomes universal, medical labeling turns into a tool for total social control. E. Richard Brown. *The Rockefeller Medicine Men: Medicine & Capitalism in the Progressive Era.* Berkeley, U. of California Press, forthcoming 1977. Demonstrates how medical tests were used for social control in Guatemala.

[259]Siegler and Osmond, "Aesculapian Authority." See p. 40 footnote 32. According to the authors, Aesculapian authority was first mentioned in T. T. Paterson, "Notes on Aesculapian Authority," unpublished manuscript, 1957. It comprises three roles: sapiential authority to advise, instruct, and direct; moral authority, which makes medical actions the right thing and not just something good; and charismatic authority, by which the doctor can appeal to some supreme power and which often outranks the patient's conscience and the *raison d'etat*. Pedagogues, psychologists, movement leaders, and nonconventional healers tend increasingly to appeal to this three-tiered authority in the name of their peculiar technique, thus joining the ranks of the scientific doctors and contributing to a cancerous expansion of the Aesculapian role.

[260]Franco Basaglia, *La maggioranza deviante: L'ideologia del controllo sociale totale,* Nuovo Politecnico no. 43 (Turin: Einaudi, 1971). Since the sixties a citizen without a medically recognized status has come to constitute an exception. A fundamental condition of contemporary political control is the conditioning of people to believe they need such a status for the sake not only of their own but of other people's health.

The role of the doctor has now become blurred.[261] The health professions have come to combine clinical service, public-health engineering, and scientific medicine. The doctor deals with clients who are simultaneously cast in several roles during every contact they have with the health establishment. They are turned into patients whom medicine tests and repairs, into administered citizens whose healthy behavior a medical bureaucracy guides, and into guinea pigs on whom medical science constantly experiments. The Aesculapian power of conferring the sick-role has been dissolved by the pretensions of delivering totalitarian health care. Health has ceased to be a native endowment each human being is presumed to possess until proven ill, and has become an ever-receding goal to which one is entitled by virtue of social justice.

The emergence of a conglomerate health profession has rendered the patient role infinitely elastic. The doctor's certification of the sick has been replaced by the bureaucratic presumption of the health manager who arranges people according to degrees and categories of therapeutic need, and medical authority now extends to supervised health care, early detection, preventive therapies, and increasingly, treatment of the incurable. Previously modern medicine controlled only a limited market; now this market has lost all boundaries. Unsick people have come to depend on professional care for the sake of their future health. The result is a morbid society that demands

---

[261]Nils Christie, "Law and Medicine: The Case Against Role Blurring," *Law and Society Review* 5 (February 1971): 357–66. A case study by a criminologist of the conflict between two monopolistic professional empires. Medicine converges with education and law enforcement. The medicalization of all diagnosis denies the deviant the right to his own values: he who accepts the patient role implies by this submission that, once restored to health (which is just a different kind of patient role in our society), he will conform. The medicalization of his complaint results in the political castration of his suffering. For this see Jesse R. Pitts, "Social Control: The Concept," *International Encyclopedia of the Social Sciences* (1968), 14:391.

universal medicalization and a medical establishment that certifies universal morbidity.

In a morbid society[262] the belief prevails that defined and diagnosed ill-health is infinitely preferable to any other form of negative label or to no label at all. It is better than criminal or political deviance, better than laziness, better than self-chosen absence from work. More and more people subconsciously know that they are sick and tired of their jobs and of their leisure passivities, but they want to hear the lie that physical illness relieves them of social and political responsibilities. They want their doctor to act as lawyer and priest. As a lawyer, the doctor exempts the patient from his normal duties and enables him to cash in on the insurance fund he was forced to build. As a priest, he becomes the patient's accomplice in creating the myth that he is an innocent victim of biological mechanisms rather than a lazy, greedy, or envious deserter of a social struggle for control over the tools of production. Social life becomes a giving and receiving of therapy: medical, psychiatric, pedagogic, or geriatric. Claiming access to treatment becomes a political duty, and medical certification a powerful device for social control.

With the development of the therapeutic service sector of the economy, an increasing proportion of all people come to be perceived as deviating from some desirable norm, and therefore as clients who can now either be submitted to therapy to bring them closer to the established standard of health or concentrated into some special environment built to cater to their deviance. Basaglia[263] points out that in the first historical stage of this process, the diseased are exempted from production. At the next stage of industrial expansion, a majority come to be defined as deviant and in need of therapy. When this happens, the distance between the sick and the healthy is again

---

[262]H. Huebschmann, "La Notion d'une société malade," *Présence,* no. 94 (1966), pp. 25–40.

[263]Basaglia, *La maggioranza deviante.*

reduced. In advanced industrial societies the sick are once more recognized as possessing a certain level of productivity which would have been denied them at an earlier stage of industrialization. Now that everybody tends to be a patient in some respect, wage labor acquires therapeutic characteristics. Lifelong health education, counseling, testing, and maintenance are built right into factory and office routine. Therapeutic dependencies permeate and color productive relations. *Homo sapiens,* who awoke to myth in a tribe and grew into politics as a citizen, is now trained as a lifelong inmate of an industrial world.[264] The medicalization of industrial society brings its imperialistic character to ultimate fruition.

---

[264] Michel Foucault, ***Surveiller et punir: Naissance de la prison*** (Paris: Gallimard, 1975). On the rise of the pan-therapeutic society in which morality-charged roles are extinguished. English translation to be published by Pantheon Books, New York.

Part III

Cultural Iatrogenesis

Introduction

We have dealt so far with two ways in which the predominance of medicalized health care becomes an obstacle to a healthy life: first, clinical iatrogenesis, which results when organic coping capacity is replaced by heteronomous management; and, second, social iatrogenesis, in which the environment is deprived of those conditions that endow individuals, families, and neighborhoods with control over their own internal states and over their milieu. Cultural iatrogenesis represents a third dimension of medical health-denial. It sets in when the medical enterprise saps the will of people to suffer their reality.[1] It is a symptom of such iatrogenesis that the term "suffering" has become almost useless for designating a realistic human response because it evokes superstition, sadomasochism, or the rich man's condescension to the lot of the poor. Professionally organized medicine has come to function as a domineering moral enterprise that advertises industrial expansion as a war against all suffering. It has thereby undermined the ability of individuals to face their reality, to express

[1]F. J. J. Buytendijk, *Allgemeine Theorie der menschlichen Haltung und Bewegung* (Berlin: Springer, 1956). Through a comparison with other species, he comes to describe man as a physiologically and psychologically self-structuring organism. For an orientation in English on the German literature in this field see H. O. Pappe, "On Philosophical Anthropology," *Australasian Journal of Philosophy* 39 (1961): 47–64.

their own values, and to accept inevitable and often irremediable pain and impairment, decline, and death.

To be in good health means not only to be successful in coping with reality but also to enjoy the success; it means to be able to feel alive in pleasure and in pain; it means to cherish but also to risk survival. Health and suffering as experienced sensations are phenomena that distinguish men from beasts.[2] Only storybook lions are said to *suffer* and only pets to merit compassion when they are in ill health.[3]

Human health adds openness to instinctual performance.[4] It is something more than a concrete behavior pattern in customs, usages, traditions, or habit-clusters. It implies performance according to a set of control mechanisms: plans, recipes, rules, and instructions, all of which govern personal behavior.[5] To a large extent culture and health coincide. Each culture gives shape to a unique *Gestalt* of health and to a unique conformation of attitudes towards pain,

---

[2]Adolf Portmann, *Zoologie und das neue Bild des Menschen* (Hamburg: Rowohlt, 1956). Man has no built-in evolutionary mechanism that would lead him to an equilibrium; his creative availability gives to his environment *(Umwelt)* characteristics different from those it has for other species: it turns habitat into home.

[3]Peter Sedgwick, "Illness, Mental and Otherwise: All Illnesses Express a Social Judgment," *Hastings Center Studies* 1, no. 3 (1973): 19–40.

[4]Viktor von Weiszäcker, *Der Gestaltkreis: Theorie der Einheit von Wahrnehmen und Bewegen,* 4th ed. (Stuttgart: Thieme, 1968; 1st ed. 1940).

[5]Henry E. Sigerist, *A History of Medicine,* vol. 1, *Primitive and Archaic Medicine* (New York: Oxford Univ. Press, 1967). Erwin H. Ackerknecht, "Primitive Medicine and Culture Patterns," *Bulletin of the History of Medicine* 12 (November 1942): 545–74. Sigerist states: "Culture, whether or not primitive, always has a certain configuration. . . . The medicine of a primitive tribe fits into that pattern. It is one expression of it, and cannot be fully understood if it is studied separately." Ackerknecht exemplifies this integration of culture and medicine in three tribes: the Cheyenne, Dobuan, and Thonga. For a classic description of this integration see E. E. Evans-Pritchard, *Witchcraft, Oracles and Magic Among the Azandé* (New York: Oxford Univ. Press, 1937), pt. 4, 3. I argue here that health and my ability to remain responsible for my behavior in suffering are correlated. Relief from this responsibility correlates with a decline in health.

disease, impairment, and death, each of which designates a class of that human performance that has traditionally been called the art of suffering.[6]

Each person's health is a responsible performance in a social script.[7] How he relates to the sweetness and the bitterness of reality and how he acts towards others whom he perceives as suffering, as weakened, or as anguished determine each person's sense of his own body, and with it, his health. Bodysense is experienced as an ever-renewed gift of culture.[8] In Java people flatly say, "To be human is to be Javanese." Small children, boors, simpletons, the insane, and the flagrantly immoral are said to be *ndurung djawa* (not yet Javanese). A "normal" adult capable of acting in terms of the highly elaborate system of etiquette, possessed of the delicate aesthetic perceptions associated with music, dance, drama, and

---

[6]It is not easy to study medical culture without a straitjacket. F. L. Dunn, "Traditional Asian Medicine and Cosmopolitan Medicine as Adaptative Systems," mimeographed, Univ. of California, n.d. Dunn indicates an important bias in most published research on medical cultures. He claims that 95% of the ethnographic (and also anthropological) literature on health-enhancing behavior and on the beliefs underlying it deals with curing and not with the maintenance and expansion of health. For literature on medical culture seen with the blinkers of the behavioral technician: Marion Pearsall, *Medical Behavioral Science: A Selected Bibliography of Cultural Anthropology, Social Psychology and Sociology in Medicine* (Lexington: Univ. of Kentucky Press, 1963). See also Steven Polgar, references in note 19, p. 8 above. Elfriede Grabner, *Volksmedizin: Probleme und Forschungsgeschichte* (Darmstadt: Wissenschaftliche Buchgesellschaft, 1974), provides an anthology of critical studies on the history of ethnomedicine.

[7]On the cultural uniqueness of health: Ina-Maria Greverus, *Der territoriale Mensch: Ein literaturanthropologischer Versuch zum Heimatphänomen* (Frankfurt: Athenäum, 1972). W. E. Muhlmann, "Das Problem der Umwelt beim Menschen," *Zeitschrift für Morphologia und Anthropologia* 44 (1952): 153–81. Arnold Gehlen, *Die Seele im technischen Zeitalter, Sozialpsychologische Probleme in der industriellen Gesellschaft* (Hamburg: Rowohlt, 1957). P. Berger, B. Berger, and H. Kellner, *The Homeless Mind* (New York: Vintage Books, 1974).

[8]Herbert Plüge, *Der Mensch und sein Leib* (Tübingen: Niemeyer, 1967). F. J. J. Buytendijk, *Mensch und Tier* (Hamburg: Rowohlt, 1958). F. J. J. Buytendijk, *Prolegomena to an Anthropological Physiology* (Pittsburgh, Pa.: Duquesne University Press, 1974).

textile design, and responsive to the subtle promptings of the divine residing in the stillness of each individual's inward-turning consciousness is *ampun djawa* (already Javanese). To be human is not just to breathe; it is also to control one's breathing by yoga-like techniques so as to hear in inhalation and exhalation the literal voice of God pronouncing his own name, *hu Allah.*[9] Cultural health is bounded by each society's style in the art of living, feasting, suffering, and dying.[10]

All traditional cultures derive their hygienic function from this ability to equip the individual with the means for making pain tolerable, sickness, or impairment understandable, and the shadow of death meaningful. In such cultures health care is always a program for eating,[11] drinking,[12] working,[13] breathing,[14] loving,[15] politicking,[16] exercising,[17] singing,[18]

---

[9]Clifford Geertz, "The Impact of the Concept of Culture on the Concept of Man," in Yehudi A. Cohen, ed., *Man in Adaptation: The Cultural Present* (Chicago: Aldine, 1968). See also Clifford Geertz, *The interpretation of culture.* Basic Books 1973. see also critique of the point of view that is here espoused in: Mary Douglas. "The self-completing animal," in: Times Literary Supplement. August 8, 1975. pp 886–887.

[10]Erwin H. Ackerknecht, "Natural Diseases and Rational Treatment in Primitive Medicine," *Bulletin of the History of Medicine* 19 (May 1946): 467–97, is a dated but still excellent review of the literature on the functions of medical cultures. Ackerknecht provides convergent evidence that medicine plays a social role and has a holistic and unitarian character in primitive cultures that modern medicine cannot provide.

[11]Hans Wiswe, *Kulturgeschichte der Kochkunst: Kochbücher und Rezepte aus zwei Jahrtausenden* (Munich: Moos, 1970). Fred Binder, *Die Brotnahrung: Auswahl-Bibliographie zu ihrer Geschichte und Bedeutung,* Donau Schriftreihe no. 9 (Ulm: Deutsches Brotmuseum E.V., 1973). Ludwig Edelstein, *Ancient Medicine: Selected Papers of Ludwig Edelstein,* C. Lilian and Owsei Temkin, eds. (Baltimore: Johns Hopkins, 1967). See the chapter on dietetics in antiquity.

[12]Salvatore P. Lucia, *Wine and the Digestive System: A Select and Annotated Bibliography* (San Francisco: Fortune House, 1970).

[13]Lucien Febvre, "Travail: Évolution d'un mot et d'une idée," *Journal de psychologie normale et pathologique* 41, no. 1 (1948): 19–28.

[14]Richard B. Onians, *The Origins of European Thought About the Body, the Mind, the Soul, the World, Time and Fate* (1951; reprinted ed., New York: Arno, 1970). H. E. Sigerist, "Disease and

dreaming,[19] warring, and suffering. Most healing is a traditional way of consoling, caring, and comforting people while they heal, and most sick-care a form of tolerance extended to the afflicted. Only those cultures survive that provide a viable code that is adapted to a group's genetic make-up, to its history, to its environment, and to the peculiar challenges represented by competing groups of neighbors.

The ideology promoted by contemporary cosmopolitan medical enterprise runs counter to these functions.[20] It radically undermines the continuation of old cultural programs and prevents the emergence of new ones that would provide a pattern for self-care and suffering. Wherever in the world a culture is medicalized, the traditional framework for habits that

---

Music," in *Civilization and Disease* (Chicago: Univ. of Chicago Press, 1943), chap. 11, pp. 212 ff.

[15]Günter Elsässer, "Ausfall des Coitus als Krankheitsursache in der Medizin des Mittelalters," in Paul Diepgen et al., eds., *Abhandlung zur Geschichte der Medizin und der Naturwissenschaften*, no. 3 (Berlin, 1934). Robert H. van Gulik, *Sexual Life in Ancient China* (Atlantic Highlands, N.J.: Humanities Press, 1961).

[16]Werner Jaeger, *Paideia: The Ideals of Greek Culture* (New York: Oxford Univ. Press, 1943), vol. 3, chap. 1, "Greek Medicine as Paideia," pp. 3–45.

[17]Edward N. Gardiner, *Athletics of the Ancient World* (New York: Oxford Univ. Press, 1930). M. Michler, "Das Problem der westgriechischen Heilkunde," *Sudhoffs Archiv* 46 (1962): 141 ff.

[18]Fridolf Kudlien, "Stimmübungen als Therapeutikum in der antiken Medizin," *Ärztliche Mitteilungen* 44 (1963): 2257–8; for a digest of this article see L. Heyer-Grote, *Atemschulung als Element der Psychotherapie* (Darmstadt: Wissenschaftliche Buchgesellschaft, 1970). Johanna Schmidt, "Phonaskoi," in Pauly-Wissowa, *Real-Encyklopädie* (1941), 20, pt. 1:522–6.

[19]A. W. Gubser, "Ist der Mittagsschlaf schädlich?" *Schweizerische Medizinische Wochenschrift* 97, no. 7 (1967): 213–16. Jane Belo, *Trance in Bali*, preface by Margaret Mead (New York: Columbia Univ. Press, 1960). Kilton Steward, "Dream Theory in Malaya," *Complex: The Magazine of Psychoanalysis and Related Matters* 6 (1951): 21–33.

[20]Ibn Khaldun, *The Muqaddimah: An Introduction to History*, trans. Franz Rosenthal, Bollingen Series XLIII, 3 vols. (Princeton, N.J.: Princeton Univ. Press, 1967). Writing towards the end of the 15th century Ibn Khaldun observed the conflict between the craft of medicine required by sedentary culture and its luxury and Bedouin medicine, which was based mainly upon tradition and individual experience. See especially 2:373–7 and 3:149–51.

can become conscious in the personal practice of the virtue of hygiene is progressively trammeled by a mechanical system, a medical code by which individuals submit to the instructions emanating from hygienic custodians.[21] Medicalization constitutes a prolific bureaucratic program based on the denial of each man's need to deal with pain, sickness, and death.[22] The modern medical enterprise represents an endeavor to do for people what their genetic and cultural heritage formerly equipped them to do for themselves. Medical civilization is planned and organized to kill pain, to eliminate sickness, and to abolish the need for an art of suffering and of dying. This progressive flattening out of personal, virtuous performance constitutes a new goal which has never before been a guideline for social life. Suffering, healing, and dying, which are essentially intransitive activities that culture taught each man, are now claimed by technocracy as new areas of policy-making and are treated as malfunctions from which populations ought to be institutionally relieved. The goals of metropolitan medical civilization are thus in opposition to

---

[21]F. N. L. Poynter, ed., *Medicine and Culture,* Proceedings of a Historical Symposium Organized Jointly by the Wellcome Institute of the History of Medicine, London, and the Wenner-Gren Foundations for Anthropological Research, N.Y. (London: Wellcome Institute, 1969). See for the conflict between metropolitan medicine and various traditions. On the use of one hospital to create the new category of "mental disease" in Senegal, see Danielle Storper-Perez, *La Folie colonisée: Textes à l'appui* (Paris: Maspero, 1974).

[22]The Western idea that *health* in the abstract is a property of man could not develop except parallel to the idea of *mankind.* Carlyle suggests that both ideas first took recognizable form in the toast of the victorious Alexander to the *homo-ousia* (like-naturedness) of men. Combined with the idea of progress, the utopia of healthy mankind came to prevail over the ideal of concrete and specific patterns of functioning characteristic for each tribe or *polis.* On this see H. C. Baldry, *The Unity of Mankind in Greek Thought* (Cambridge: University Press, 1965), and Max Muehl, *Die antike Menschheitsidee in ihrer geschichtlichen Entwicklung* (Leipzig: Dietrichsche Verlagsbuchhandlung, 1928). Sidney Pollard, *The Idea of Progress: History and Society* (New York: Basic Books, 1968), deals with the ideology of *human progress* in relation to concrete history and the politico-economic aspects complementing philosophy.

every single cultural health program they encounter in the process of progressive colonization.[23]

---

[23]To study this clash in Latin American history, see, on ethnomedicine, Erwin H. Ackerknecht, "Medical Practices," in Julian Haynes Steward, *Handbook of South American Indians,* vol. 5, *The Comparative Ethnology of South American Indians* (1949; reprinted ed., Saint Clair Shores, Mich.; Scholarly Press, 1973), pp. 625–43. On medical colonization, see Percy M. Ashburn, *The Ranks of Death: A Medical History of the Conquest of America* (New York: Coward-McCann, 1947). An important work, throwing light on the history of medicine and on the conquest. Francisco Guerra, *Historiografía de la medicina colonial hispano-americana* (Mexico: Abastecedora de impresos, 1953), is more bibliographical than historiographical, but indispensable. No comprehensive study of the imperialism of European medical ideology in Latin America is available. For a first orientation, see Gonzalo Aguirre Beltrán, *Medicina y magia: El proceso de aculturación en la estructura colonial* (Mexico: Instituto Nacional Indigenista, 1963). Rudolf Thissen, Die Entwicklung der Terminologie auf dem Gebiet der Sozialhygiene und Sozialmedizin im deutschen Sprachgebiet bis 1930. Forschungsbericht des Landes Nordrhein-Westfalen. Nr 2050. Köln, Westdeutscher Verlag, 1969. pp. 3–72. A history of the terms used in social medicine since hygiene in Germany passed from the control of the clergy to that of the physician. Particularly illuminating on the mid-19th century, when health became the "only property" of the worker, that had to be protected by government action.

3

The Killing of Pain

When cosmopolitan medical civilization colonizes any traditional culture, it transforms the experience of pain.[1] The same nervous stimulation that I shall call "pain sensation" will result in a distinct experience, depending not only on personality but also on culture. This experience, as distinct from the painful sensation, implies a uniquely human performance called *suffering*.[2] Medical civilization, however, tends to turn pain into a technical matter and thereby deprives suffering of its inherent personal meaning.[3] People unlearn the acceptance of suffering as an inevitable part of their conscious coping with reality

---

[1]For a very sensitive phenomenological analysis of the modernization of the pain experience, see Peter Berger, "Policy and the Calculus of Pain," in *Pyramids of Sacrifice: Political Ethics and Social Change* (New York: Basic Books, 1974), chap. 5.

[2]F. J. J. Buytendijk, *Pain, Its Modes and Functions,* trans. Eda O'Shiel (Chicago: Univ. of Chicago Press, 1962). Rudolf Bilz, *Paläoanthropologie,* vols. 1–2, *Studien über Angst und Schmerz* (Frankfurt am Main: Suhrkamp, 1971).

[3]Victor Weizsäcker, *Arzt und Kranker* (Stuttgart: Köhler, 1949), vol. 1.

and learn to interpret every ache as an indicator of their need for padding or pampering. Traditional cultures confront pain, impairment, and death by interpreting them as challenges soliciting a response from the individual under stress; medical civilization turns them into demands made by individuals on the economy, into problems that can be managed or *produced* out of existence.[4] Cultures are systems of meanings, cosmopolitan civilization a system of techniques. Culture makes pain tolerable by integrating it into a meaningful setting; cosmopolitan civilization detaches pain from any subjective or intersubjective context in order to annihilate it. Culture makes pain tolerable by interpreting its necessity; only pain perceived as curable is intolerable.

A myriad virtues express the different aspects of fortitude that traditionally enabled people to recognize painful sensations as a challenge and to shape their own experience accordingly. Patience, forbearance, courage, resignation, self-control, perseverance, and meekness each express a different coloring of the responses with which pain sensations were accepted, transformed into the experience of suffering, and endured.[5] Duty, love, fascination, routines, prayer, and compassion were some of the means that enabled pain to be borne with dignity. Traditional cultures made everyone responsible for his own performance under the impact of bodily harm or grief.[6] Pain was recog-

---

[4]Thomas S. Szasz, *Pain and Pleasure* (New York: Basic Books, 1957).

[5]For an analysis of the reaction to pain on the part of contemporary authors and philosophers, see Ida Cermak, *Ich klage nicht: Begegnungen mit der Krankheit in Selbstzeugnissen schöpferischer Menschen* (Vienna: Amalthea, 1972). In late medieval times it was almost impossible to recognize, from the behavior of a person in pain, if the origin of the experience was grief, compassion, hurt pride, or a wound. Wilhelm Scherer, *Der Ausdruck des Schmerzes und der Freude in der mittelhochdeutschen Dichtung der Blütezeit* (Strassburg, 1908).

[6]When the artists of classical Greece portrayed pain, they were only indirectly concerned with its physiological impact and principally tried to represent the more or less personal way this impact was experienced. Ernst Hannes Brauer, *Studien zur Darstellung des Schmerzes in der antiken bildenden Kunst Griechenlands und Italiens,*

nized as an inevitable part of the subjective reality of one's own body in which everyone constantly finds himself, and which is constantly being shaped by his conscious reactions to it.[7] People knew that they had to heal on their own,[8] to deal on their own with their migraine, their lameness, or their grief.

The pain inflicted on individuals had a limiting effect on the abuses of man by man. Exploiting minorities sold liquor or preached religion to dull their victims, and slaves took to the blues or to coca-chewing. But beyond a critical point of exploitation, traditional economies which were built on the resources of the human body had to break down. Any society in which the intensity of discomforts and pains inflicted rendered them culturally "insufferable" could not but come to an end.

Now an increasing portion of all pain is man-made, a side-effect of strategies for industrial expansion. Pain has ceased to be conceived as a "natural" or "metaphysical" evil. It is a social curse, and to stop the "masses" from cursing society when they are pain-stricken, the industrial system delivers them medical pain-killers. Pain thus turns into a demand for more drugs, hospitals, medical services, and other outputs of corporate, impersonal care and into politi-

---

inaugural dissertation, Univ. of Breslau (Breslau: Nischkowsky, 1934). For analogous conclusions about the Attic theater, Karl Kiefer, *Körperlicher Schmerz auf der attischen Bühne,* inaugural dissertation (Heidelberg: Carl Winter's Universitätsbuchhandlung, 1908).

[7]For 60 plastic representations of human beings in pain, see Friedrich Schulze-Maizier and H. Moehle, *Schmerz* (Berlin: Metzner, 1943). Also F. Garnaud, "La Douleur dans l'art," *Aesculape,* 1957, several pages in successive issues.

[8]Victor Weiszäcker, "Zum Begriff der Arbeit: Eine Habeas-Corpus Akte der Medizin?" in Edgar Salin, ed., *Synopsis: Festgabe für Alfred Weber* (Heidelberg: Schneider, 1948), pp. 707–61. A phenomenological description of suffering as a *Leistung,* i.e., an activity of the sick person which elicits respect in all societies and is usually recognized as a "performance" that, though different from work, has a social status analogous to it. Albert Görres, ed., *Der Kranke, Ärgernis der Leistungsgesellschaft* (Düsseldorf: Patmos, 1971). Although he does not go that far, Everett Hughes, *Men and Their Work* (New York: Free Press, 1958), provides a basis for a similar interpretation.

cal support for further corporate growth no matter what its human, social, or economic cost. Pain has become a political issue which gives rise to a snowballing demand on the part of anesthesia consumers for artificially induced insensibility, unawareness, and even unconsciousness.

Traditional cultures and technological civilization start from opposite assumptions. In every traditional culture the psychotherapy, belief systems, and drugs needed to withstand most pain are built into everyday behavior and reflect the conviction that reality is harsh and death inevitable.[9] In the twentieth century dystopia, the necessity to bear painful reality, within or without, is interpreted as a failure of the socioeconomic system, and pain is treated as an emergent contingency which must be dealt with by extraordinary interventions.

The experience of pain that results from pain messages received by the brain depends in its quality and in its quantity on genetic endowment[10] and on at least four functional factors other than the nature and intensity of the stimulus: namely, culture, anxiety, attention, and interpretation. All these are shaped by social determinants, ideology, economic structure, and social character. Culture decrees whether the mother or the father or both must groan when the child is born.[11] Circumstances and habits determine the anxiety level of the sufferer and the attention he

---

[9]Bilz, "Die Menschheitsgeschichtlich ältesten Mythologeme," in *Studien über Angst und Schmerz,* pp. 276–94.

[10]Asenath Petrie, *Individuality in Pain and Suffering* (Chicago: Univ. of Chicago Press, 1967). People differ in the intensity with which they modulate experience; some reduce and others increase what is perceived, including pain. This reaction pattern is partially determined genetically. See also B. B. Wolff and M. E. Jarvik, "Relationship Between Superficial and Deep Somatic Threshold of Pain, with a Note on Handedness," *American Journal of Psychology* 77 (1964): 589–99.

[11]For the person who is supposed to suffer at childbirth, and the place in the body where pain is supposed to originate, see Grantly Dick-Read, *Childbirth Without Fear* (1944; paperback ed., New York: Dell, 1962). Contains much information on the impact of culture on the level of fear and the relationship between fear and the pain experience.

gives to his bodily sensations.[12] Training and conviction determine the meaning given to bodily sensations and influence the degree to which pain is experienced.[13] Effective magic relief is often better provided by popular superstition than by high-class religion.[14] The prospect which is opened by the painful event determines how well it will be suffered: injuries received near the climax of sex or that of heroic performance are frequently not even felt. Soldiers wounded on the Anzio Beachhead who hoped their wounds would get them out of the army and back home as heroes rejected morphine injections that they would have considered absolutely necessary if similar injuries had been inflicted by the dentist or in the operating theater.[15]

As culture is medicalized, the social determinants of pain are distorted. Whereas culture recognizes pain

---

[12]Henry K. Beecher, *Measurement of Subjective Responses: Quantitative Effects of Drugs* (New York: Oxford Univ. Press, 1959). Opiates exert their principal action, not on the pain impulse, which is transmitted through the nervous system, but on the psychological overlay of pain. They lower the level of anxiety. Placebos can achieve the same effect in many people. Severe postsurgical pain can be relieved in about 35% of patients by giving them a sugar or saline tablet instead of an analgesic. Since only 75% are relieved under such circumstances with large doses of morphine, the placebo effect might account for 50% of drug effectiveness. See also Harris Hill et al., "Studies on Anxiety Associated with Anticipation of Pain: I. Effects of Morphine," *A.M.A. Archives of Neurology and Psychiatry* 67 (May 1952): 612–19.

[13]R. Melzack and T. H. Scott, "The Effect of Early Experience on the Response to Pain," *Journal of Comparative and Physiological Psychology* 50 (April 1957): 155–61. For a phenomenological analysis see Victor E. von Gebsattel, *Imago hominis: Beiträge zu einer personalen Anthropologie,* 2nd ed. (Salzburg: Otto Müller, 1968); Jacques Sarano, *La Douleur* (Lyons: Editions de l'Epi, 1965).

[14]Thomas Keith, *Religion and the Decline of Magic: Studies in Popular Beliefs in the 16th and 17th Centuries in England* (London: Weidenfeld, 1971). On the importance and practical utility of religion and superstition in early modern England in the relief of suffering.

[15]Beecher, *Measurement of Subjective Responses,* pp. 164 ff. Howard S. Becker, "Consciousness, power and drug effects." in: Journal of Psychedelic Drugs, Vol. 6, No. 1, Jan.–Mar., 1974. pp. 67–76. Drug effects vary greatly, depending on variations in the user's ideas and beliefs about the drug, and on the control he exercises over the use of the drug.

as an intrinsic, intimate, and incommunicable "disvalue," medical civilization focuses primarily on pain as a systemic reaction that can be verified, measured, and regulated. Only pain perceived by a third person from a distance constitutes a diagnosis that calls for specific treatment. This objectivization and quantification of pain goes so far that medical treatises speak of painful diseases, operations, or conditions even in cases where patients claim to be unaware of pain. Pain calls for methods of control by the physician rather than an approach that might help the person in pain take on responsibility for his experience.[16] The medical profession judges which pains are authentic, which have a physical and which a psychic base, which are imagined, and which are simulated.[17] Society recognizes and endorses this professional judgment. Compassion becomes an obsolete virtue. The person in pain is left with less and less social context to give meaning to the experience that often overwhelms him.

The history of medical perception of pain has not yet been written. A few learned monographs deal with the moments during the last 250 years in which the attitude of physicians towards pain changed,[18] and some historical references can be found in papers dealing with contemporary attitudes towards pain.[19]

---

[16]For information on this subject consult James D. Hardy et al., *Pain Sensations and Reactions* (1952; reprint ed., New York: Hafner, 1967); Harold G. and Stewart Wolff, *Pain*, American Lectures in Physiology Series, 2nd ed. (Springfield, Ill.: Thomas, 1958); Benjamin L. Crue, *Pain and Suffering: Selected Aspects* (Springfield, Ill.: Thomas, 1970).

[17]Thomas S. Szasz, "The Psychology of Persistent Pain: A Portrait of L'Homme Douloureux," in A. Soulairac, J. Cahn, and J. Charpentier, eds., *Pain* (New York: Academic Press, 1968), pp. 93–113.

[18]Richard Toellner, "Die Umbewertung des Schmerzes im 17. Jahrhundert in ihren Vorraussetzungen und Folgen," *Medizinhistorisches Journal* 6 (1971): 707–61. Ferdinand Sauerbruch and Hans Wenke, *Wesen und Bedeutung des Schmerzes* (Berlin: Junker & Dünnhaupt, 1936). Thomas Keys, *History of Surgical Anesthesia*, rev. ed. (New York: Dover, 1963).

[19]Kenneth D. Keele, *Anatomies of Pain* (Springfield, Ill.: Thomas, 1957). Hermann Buddensieg, *Leid und Schmerz als Schöpfermacht* (Heidelberg: n.p., 1956).

The existential school of anthropological medicine has gathered valuable insights into the development of modern pain while tracing the changes in bodily perception in a technological age.[20] The relationship between the medical institutions and the anxiety suffered by their patients has been explored by psychiatrists[21] and occasionally by general physicians. But the relationship of corporate medicine to bodily pain in its real sense is still virgin territory for research.

The historian of pain has to face three special problems. The first is the profound transformation undergone by the relationship of pain to the other ills man can suffer. Pain has changed its position in relation to grief, guilt, sin, anguish, fear, hunger, impairment, and discomfort. What we call pain in a surgical ward is something for which former generations had no special name. It now seems as if pain were only that part of human suffering over which the medical profession can claim competence or control. There is no historical precedent for the contemporary situation in which the experience of personal bodily pain is shaped by the therapeutic program designed to destroy it.

The second problem is language. The technical matter which contemporary medicine designates by the term "pain" even today has no simple equivalent in ordinary speech. In most languages the term taken over by the doctors covers grief, sorrow, anguish, shame, and guilt. The English "pain" and the German "Schmerz" are still relatively easy to use in such a

---

[20]Gebsattel, *Imago hominis.* Sarano, *La Douleur.* Karl E. Rothschuh, *Physiologie: Der Wandel ihrer Konzepte, Probleme und Methoden vom 16. bis 20. Jahrhundert* (Freiburg: Alber, 1968). An invaluable guide to the history of physiology since the 16th century, which comes as close as possible to a history of the medical perception of pain. Karl E. Rothschuh, *Von Boerhaave bis Berger: Die Entwicklung der kontinentalen Psychologie im 18. und 19. Jahrhundert mit besonderer Beruecksichtigung der Neurophysiologie* (Stuttgart: Fischer, 1964).

[21]H. Merskey and F. G. Spear, *Pain: Psychological and Psychiatric Aspects* (London: Bailliere, Tindall & Cassell, 1967), reviews significant papers and attempts a clarification of the use of pain in experimental work.

way that a mostly, though not exclusively, physical meaning is conveyed. Most Indo-Germanic synonyms cover a wider range of meaning:[22] bodily pain may be designated as "hard work," "toil," or "trial," as "torture," "endurance," "punishment," or more generally, "affliction," as "illness," "tiredness," "hunger," "mourning," "injury," "distress," "sadness," "trouble," "confusion," or "oppression." This litany is far from complete: it shows that language can distinguish many kinds of "evils," all of which have a bodily reflection. In some languages bodily pain is outright "evil." If a French doctor asks a typical Frenchman where he has pain, the patient will point to the spot and say, "J'ai mal là." On the other hand, a Frenchman can say, "Je souffre dans toute ma chair," and at the same time tell his doctor, "Je n'ai mal nulle part." If the concept of bodily pain has undergone an evolution in medical usage, it cannot be grasped simply in the changing significance of any one term.

A third obstacle to any history of pain is its exceptional axiological and epistemological status.[23] Nobody will ever understand "my pain" in the way I

---

[22]See Carl Darling Buck, *A Dictionary of Selected Synonyms in the Principal Indo-European Languages: A Contribution to the History of Ideas* (Chicago: Univ. of Chicago Press, 1949), for the following four semantic fields: pain-suffering, 16.31; grief-sorrow, 16.32; emotion-feeling, 16.12; passion, 16.13. See also W. Frenzen, *Klagebilder und Klagegebärden in der deutschen Dichtung des höfischen Mittelalters,* dissertation, Univ. of Bonn (Würzburg: Triltsch, 1938). Georg Zappert, "Über den Ausdruck des geistigen Schmerzes im Mittelalter: Ein Beitrag zur Geschichte der Förderungs-Momente des Rührenden im Romantischen," in *Denkschriften der Kaiserlichen Akademie der Wissenschaften* (Vienna: Philosophisch-historisch Classe, 1854), 5: 73–136.

[23]Robert S. Hartman, *The Structure of Value: Foundation of Scientific Axiology* (Carbondale: Southern Illinois Univ. Press, 1967), especially pp. 255 ff. A distinction is made between "my pain," an intrinsic disvalue about which a totally unique certainty exists; "your pain," an extrinsic disvalue for which I can experience compassion; and "the kind of pain from which a third person is said to suffer," such as the migraines of unspecified patients, for which I can at best solicit some general sympathy. The pain about which a history ought to be written is the personalized experience of intrinsic pain: the inclusion in the experience of pain of the social situation in which pain occurs.

mean it, unless he suffers the same headache, which is impossible, because he is another person. In this sense "pain" means a breakdown of the clear-cut distinction between organism and environment, between stimulus and response.[24] It does not mean a certain class of experience that allows you and me to compare our headaches; much less does it mean a certain physiological or medical entity, a clinical case with certain pathological signs. It is not "pain in the sternocleidomastoid" which is perceived as a systematic disvalue for the medical scientist.

The exceptional kind of disvalue that is pain promotes an exceptional kind of certainty. Just as "my pain" belongs in a unique way only to me, so I am utterly alone with it. I cannot share it. I have no doubt about the reality of the pain experience, but I cannot really tell anybody what I experience. I surmise that others have "their" pains, even though I cannot percieve what they mean when they tell me about them. I am certain about the existence of their pain only in the sense that I am certain of my compassion for them. And yet, the deeper my compassion, the deeper is my certitude about the other person's utter loneliness in relation to his experience. Indeed, I recognize the signs made by someone who is in pain, even when this experience is beyond my aid or comprehension. This awareness of extreme loneliness is a peculiarity of the compassion we feel for bodily pain; it also sets this experience apart from any other experience, from compassion for the anguished, sorrowful, aggrieved, alien, or crippled. In an extreme way, the sensation of bodily pain lacks the distance between cause and experience found in other forms of suffering.

Notwithstanding the inability to communicate

---

[24]David Bakan, *Disease, Pain and Sacrifice: Toward a Psychology of Suffering* (Boston: Beacon Press, 1968), deals with pain as a breakdown of *telos* and of *distality*. "Pain, having no other locus but the conscious ego, is almost literally the price man pays for the possession of a conscious ego . . . unless there is an awake and conscious organism, there is nothing one can sensibly refer to as pain."

bodily pain, perception of it in another is so fundamentally human that it cannot be put into parentheses. The patient cannot conceive that his doctor is unaware of his pain, any more than the man on the rack can conceive this about his torturer. The certainty that we share the experience of pain is of a very special kind, greater than the certainty that we share humanity with others. There have been people who have treated their slaves as chattels, yet recognized that this chattel was able to *suffer* pain. Slaves are more than dogs, who can be hurt but cannot suffer. Wittgenstein has shown that our special, radical certainty about the existence of pain in other people can coexist with an inextricable difficulty in explaining how this sharing of the unique can come about.[25]

It is my thesis that bodily pain, experienced as an intrinsic, intimate, and incommunicable disvalue, includes in our awareness the social situation in which those who suffer find themselves. The character of the society shapes to some degree the personality of those who suffer and thus determines the way they experience their own physical aches and hurts as concrete pain. In this sense, it should be possible to investigate the progressive transformation of the pain experience that has accompanied the medicalization of society. The act of suffering pain always has a historical dimension.

When I suffer pain, I am aware that a question is being raised. The history of pain can best be studied by focusing on that question. No matter if the pain is my own experience or if I see the gestures of another telling me that he is in pain, a question mark is written into this perception. Such a query is as integral to physical pain as the loneliness of pain. Pain is the sign for something not answered; it refers to something open, something that goes on the next moment to demand, What is wrong? How much longer? Why must I/ought I/should I/can I/suffer? Why does this kind of evil exist, and why does it strike just

---

[25] Ludwig Wittgenstein, *Philosophical Investigations* (Oxford: Oxford Univ. Press, 1953), pp. 89 ff.

me? Observers who are blind to this referential aspect of pain are left with nothing but conditioned reflexes. They are studying a guinea pig, not a human being. A physician, were he able to erase this value-loaded question shining through a patient's complaints, might recognize pain as the symptom of a specific bodily disorder, but he would not come close to the suffering that drove the patient to seek help. The development of this capacity to objectify pain is one of the results of overintensive education for physicians. By his training the physician is often enabled to focus on those aspects of a person's bodily pain that are accessible to management by outsiders: the peripheral-nerve stimulation, the transmission, the reaction to the stimulus, or even the anxiety level of the patient. Concern is limited to the management of the systemic entity, which is the only matter open to operational verification.

The personal performance of suffering escapes such experimental control and is therefore neglected in most experiments that are conducted on pain. Animals are usually used to test the "pain-killing" effects of pharmacological or surgical interventions. Once the results of animal tests have been tabulated, their validity is verified in people. Painkillers usually give more or less comparable results in guinea pigs and humans, provided those humans are used as experimental subjects and under experimental conditions similar to those under which the animals were tested. As soon as the same interventions are applied to people who are actually sick or have been wounded, the effects of the drugs are completely out of line with those found in the experimental situation. In the laboratory people feel exactly like mice. When their own life becomes painful, they usually cannot help suffering, well or badly, even when they want to respond like mice.[26]

---

[26] A. Soulairac, J. Cahn, and J. Charpentier, eds. *Pain*. Proceedings of the International Symposium Organized by the Laboratory of Psychophysiology, Faculté des Sciences, Paris, April 11–13, 1967 (New York: Academic Press, 1968), especially pp. 119–230.

Living in a society that values anesthesia, both doctors and their potential clients are retrained to smother pain's intrinsic question mark. The question raised by intimately experienced pain is transformed into a vague anxiety that can be submitted to treatment. Lobotomized patients provide the extreme example of this expropriation of pain: they "adjust at the level of domestic invalids or household pets."[27] The lobotomized person still perceives pain but he has lost the capacity to suffer from it; the experience of pain is reduced to a discomfort with a clinical name.

For an experience of pain to constitute suffering in the full sense, it must fit into a cultural framework.[28] To enable individuals to transform bodily pain into a personal experience, any culture provides at least four interrelated subprograms: words, drugs, myths, and models. Pain is shaped by culture into a question that can be expressed in words, cries, and gestures, which are often recognized as desperate attempts to share the utter confused loneliness in which pain is experienced: Italians groan and Prussians grind their teeth.

Each culture also provides its own psychoactive pharmacopeia, with customs that designate the circumstances in which drugs may be taken and the accompanying ritual.[29] Muslin Rayputs prefer alcohol and Brahmins marijuana,[30] though they intermingle in the same villages of western India.[31] Peyote is safe

---

[27]See Szasz, "Psychology of Persistent Pain."

[28]Mark Zborowski, "Cultural Components in Responses to Pain," in E. Gartly Jaco, *Patients, Physicians and Illness* (New York: Free Press, 1958), pp. 256–68.

[29]B. Holmstedt, "Historical Survey," in *Ethnopharmacologic Search for Psychoactive Drugs* (Washington, D.C.: National Institute of Mental Health, 1967), pp. 3–31.

[30]For alcohol in general, see Salvatore P. Lucia, *A History of Wine as Therapy* (New York: McGraw-Hill, 1963). Illustrates the social functions of alcohol as an intoxicant. E. R. Bloomquist, *Marihuana* (Beverly Hills, Calif.: Glencoe Press, 1968). On the setting and distribution of marijuana use since antiquity.

[31]G. M. Carstairs, "Daru and Bhang, Cultural Factors in the Choice of Intoxicant," *Quarterly Journal of Studies on Alcohol* 15 (June 1954): 220–37.

for Navajos[32] and mushrooms for the Huicholes,[33] while Peruvian highlanders have learned to survive with coca.[34] Man has not only evolved with the ability to *suffer* his pain, but also with the skills to manage it:[35] poppy growing[36] during the middle Stone Age probably preceded the planting of grains. Massage, acupuncture, and analgesic incense were known from the dawn of history.[37] Religious and mythic rationales for pain have appeared in all cultures: for the Muslims it is Kismet,[38] god-willed destiny; for the Hindus, karma,[39] a burden from past incarnation; for the Christians, a sanctifying backlash

---

[32]Robert L. Bergman, "Navajo Peyote Use: Its Apparent Safety," *American Journal of Psychiatry* 128 (December 1971): 695–9. When peyote is used in a ritual setting by members of the Native American Church, less than one bad trip occurs for every 10,000 doses taken. W. La Barre, *The Peyote Cult* (Hamden, Conn.: Shoestring Press, 1964). A thorough history of peyote use among the American Indians, including an extensive bibliography.

[33]R. G. Wasson, *Soma: Divine Mushroom of Immortality* (New York: Harcourt Brace, 1969).

[34]H. Blyed-Prieto, "Coca Leaf and Cocaine Addiction: Some Historical Notes," *Canadian Medical Association Journal* 93 (1965): 700–4. Sociological and historical information.

[35]Robert Burton, *The Anatomy of Melancholy*, 3 vols. (New York: Dutton, 1964; orig. ed. 1621). The classic treatise on Renaissance chemotherapy, which "elevates the mind from the depths of despair" by means of poppy, henbane, mandrake, nightshade, nutmeg, etc.

[36]"Opium," in *Encyclopedia Britannica* (1911), 20:130–7. The historical geography of poppy-growing and the history of its use presented in a Victorian perspective.

[37]Peter Graystone, *Acupuncture and Pain Theory: A Comprehensive Bibliography* (Vancouver: Biomedical Engineering Services, 1975). Complement with Billy and Miriam Tam, *Acupuncture: An International Bibliography* (Metuchen, N.J.: Scarecrow Press, 1973).

[38]For bibliography consult W. Montgomery Watt, *Free Will and Predestination in Early Islam* (London: Luzac, 1948). See also Duncan B. Macdonald, *Religious Attitude and Life in Islam* (1909; reprint ed., New York: AMS Press, 1969).

[39]H. H. Rowley, *Submission in Suffering and Other Essays on Eastern Thought* (Cardiff: Univ. of Wales Press, 1951). E. M. Hoch, "Bhaya, Shoka, Moha: Angst, Leid und Verwirrung in den alten indischen Schriften und ihre Bedeutung für die Entstehung von Krankheiten," in Wilhelm Bitter, ed., *Abendländische Therapie und östliche Weisheit* (Stuttgart: Klett, 1968).

of sin.[40] Finally, cultures always have provided an example on which behavior in pain could be modeled: the Buddha, the saint, the warrior, or the victim. The duty to suffer in their guise distracts attention from otherwise all-absorbing sensation and challenges the sufferer to bear torture with dignity. The cultural setting not only provides the grammar and technique, the myths and examples used in its characteristic "craft of suffering well," but also the instructions on how to integrate this repertoire. The medicalization of pain, on the other hand, has fostered a hypertrophy of just one of these modes—management by technique—and reinforced the decay of the others. Above all, it has rendered either incomprehensible or shocking the idea that skill in the art of suffering might be the most effective and universally acceptable way of dealing with pain. Medicalization deprives any culture of the integration of its program for dealing with pain.

Society not only determines how doctor and patient meet, but also what each of them shall think, feel, and do about pain. As long as the doctor conceived of himself primarily as a healer, pain assumed the role of a step towards the restoration of health. Where the doctor could not heal, he felt no qualms about telling his patient to use analgesics and thus moderate inevitable suffering. Like Oliver Wendell Holmes, the good doctor who knew that nature provided better remedies for pain than medicine could say "[with the exception of] opium, which the Creator himself seems to prescribe, for we often see the scarlet poppy growing in the cornfields as if it were foreseen that wherever there is hunger to be fed there must also be pain to be soothed; [with the exception of] a few specifics which our doctor's art did not discover; [with the exception of] wine, which is a food, and the vapours which produce the miracle of anaesthesia . . . I firmly believe that if the whole

---

[40]John Ferguson, *The Place of Suffering* (Cambridge: Clarke, 1972). A dense history of the classical and Hebrew background against which the Christian attitude towards suffering developed.

materia medica, as now used, could be sunk to the bottom of the sea, it would be all the better for mankind—and all the worse for the fishes."[41]

The ethos of the healer gave the physician the capacity for the same dignified failure for which religion, folklore, and free access to analgesics had trained the common man.[42] The functionary of contemporary medicine is in a different position: his first orientation is treatment, not healing. He is geared, not to recognize the question marks that pain raises in him who suffers, but to degrade these pains into a list of complaints that can be collected in a dossier. He prides himself on the knowledge of pain mechanics and thus escapes the patient's invitation to compassion.

One source of European attitudes towards pain certainly lies in ancient Greece. The pupils of Hippocrates[43] distinguished many kinds of disharmony, each of which caused its own kind of pain. Pain thus became a useful tool for diagnosis. It revealed to the physician which harmony the patient had to recover. Pain might disappear in the process of healing, but this was certainly not the primary object of the doctor's treatment. Whereas the Chinese tried very early to treat sickness through the removal of pain, nothing of this sort was prominent in the classical West. The Greeks did not even think about enjoying happiness without taking pain in their stride. Pain was the soul's experience of evolution. The human body was part of an irreparably impaired universe, and the sentient soul of man postulated by Aristotle was fully coextensive with his body. In this scheme there was no need to distinguish between the sense and the

---

[41]Oliver Wendell Holmes, *Medical Essays* (Boston, 1883).

[42]Jacques Sarano, "L'Échec et le médecin," in Jean Lacroix, ed., *Les Hommes devant l'échec* (Paris: PUF, 1968), chap. 3, pp. 69–81.

[43]For an exhaustive study of the diagnostic value ascribed to pain in Hippocratic literature, see A. Souques, "La Douleur dans les livres hippocratiques: Diagnostiques rétrospectifs," *Bulletin de la Société Française de l'Histoire de Médecine* 31 (1937): 209–14, 279–309; 32 (1938): 178–86; 33 (1939): 37–8, 131–44; 34 (1940): 53–9, 79–93.

experience of pain. The body had not yet been divorced from the soul, nor had sickness been divorced from pain. All words that indicated bodily pain were equally applicable to the suffering of the soul.

In view of that heritage, it would be a grave mistake to believe that resignation to pain is due exclusively to Jewish or Christian influence. Thirteen distinct Hebrew words were translated by a single Greek term for "pain" when two hundred Jews of the second century B.C. translated the Old Testament into Greek.[44] Whether or not pain for the Jew was considered an instrument of divine punishment, it was always a curse.[45] No suggestion of pain as a desirable experience can be found in the Scriptures or the Talmud.[46] It is true that specific organs were affected by pain, but those organs were conceived of also as seats of very specific emotions; the category of modern medical pain is totally alien to the Hebrew text. In the New Testament, pain is considered to be intimately entwined with sin.[47] While for the classical Greek pain had to accompany pleasure, for the Christian pain was a consequence of his commitment to joy.[48] No culture or tradition holds a monopoly on realistic resignation.

---

[44]For the evolution of the terms used to designate bodily pain and suffering in the Bible, see Gerhard Kittel, *Theologisches Wörterbuch zum Neuen Testament* (Stuttgart: Kohlhammer, 1933), the following articles: *lype* (Bultmann); *asthenés* (Stahlin); *pascho* (Michaelis); *nosos* (Oepke).

[45]Immanuel Jakobovitz, "Attitude to Pain," in *Jewish Medical Ethics* (New York: Bloch, 1967), p. 103.

[46]Julius Preuss, *Biblisch-talmudische Medizin: Beitrag zur Geschichte der Heilkunde und der Kultur überhaupt*, 3rd ed. (Berlin: Karger, 1923). Friedrich Weinreb, *Vom Sinn des Erkrankens* (Zürich: Origo, 1974): the Hebrew word for "sickness" has the same root as the word for "ordinary."

[47]Friedrich Fenner, *Die Krankheit im Neuen Testament: Eine religiöse- und medizinge-schichtliche Untersuchung*, Untersuchungen zum Neuen Testament, no. 18, 1930 (dissertation, Univ. of Jena, 1930).

[48]Harold Rowley, *Servant of the Lord and Other Essays on the Old Testament*, 2nd ed. (Naperville, Ill.: Allenson, 1965). Christopher R. North, *Suffering Servant in Deutero-Isaiah: An Historical and Critical Study*, 2nd ed. (New York: Oxford Univ. Press, 1956).

The history of pain in European culture would have to trace more than these classical and Semitic roots to find the ideologies that supported personal acceptance of pain. For the Neo-Platonist, pain was interpreted as the result of some deficiency in the celestial hierarchy. For the Manichaean, it was the result of positive malpractice on the part of an evil demiurge or creator. For the Christian, it was the loss of original integrity produced by Adam's sin. But no matter how much these religions opposed each other on dogma and morals, all of them saw pain as the bitter taste of cosmic evil, the manifestation of nature's weakness, of a diabolical will, or of a well-deserved divine curse. This attitude towards pain is a unifying and distinctive characteristic of Mediterranean postclassical cultures which lasted until the seventeenth century. As an alchemic doctor put it in the sixteenth century, pain is the "bitter tincture added to the sparkling brew of the world's seed." Each person was born with the call to learn to live in a vale of pain. The Neo-Platonist interpreted bitterness as a lack of perfection, the Cathar as disfigurement, the Christian as a wound for which he was held responsible. In dealing with the fullness of life, which found one of its major expressions in pain, people were able to stand up in heroic defiance or stoically deny the need for alleviation; they could welcome the opportunity for purification, penance, or sacrifice, and reluctantly tolerate the inevitable while seeking to relieve it. Opium, acupuncture, or hypnosis, always in combination with language, ritual, and myth, was applied to the unique human performance of *suffering pain.* One approach to pain was, however, unthinkable, at least in the European tradition: the belief that pain ought not to be suffered, alleviated, and interpreted by the person affected, but that it should be—ideally always—destroyed through the intervention of a priest, politician, or physician.

There were three reasons why the idea of professional, technical pain-killing was alien to all European civilizations.[49] First: pain was man's experience of a marred universe, not a mechanical dysfunction in one of its subsystems. The meaning of pain was cosmic and mythic, not individual and technical. Second: pain was a sign of corruption in nature, and man himself was a part of that whole. One could not be rejected without the other; pain could not be thought of as distinct from the ailment. The doctor could soften the pangs, but to eliminate the need to suffer would have meant to do away with the patient. Third: pain was an experience of the soul, and this soul was present all over the body. Pain was a non-mediated experience of evil. There could be no source of pain distinct from pain that was suffered.[50]

The campaign against pain as a personal matter to be understood and suffered got under way only when body and soul were divorced by Descartes. He constructed an image of the body in terms of geometry, mechanics, or watchmaking, a machine that could be repaired by an engineer. The body became an apparatus owned and managed by the soul, but from an almost infinite distance. The living body experience which the French refer to as "la chair" and the Germans as "der Leib" was reduced to a mechanism that the soul could inspect.[51]

For Descartes pain became a signal with which the body reacts in self-defense to protect its mechanical integrity. These reactions to danger are transmitted to the soul, which recognizes them as painful. Pain was reduced to a useful learning device: it now taught the soul how to avoid further damage to the body. Leibnitz sums up this new perspective when he quotes with approval a sentence by Regis, who was in turn a pupil of Descartes: "The great engineer of the

---

[49]See references in note 18, p. 134 above.

[50]K. E. Rothschuh, "Geschichtliches zur Physiologie des Schmerzes," in *Documenta Geigy: Problems of Pain* (Basel, 1965), p. 4. Pain was understood to be "perceived through the sensory faculty of the *sentiens anima;* [it was] conceived as a property of the soul, a property distributed through the entire body."

[51]Herbert Plüge, *Der Mensch und sein Leib* (Tübingen: Niemeyer, 1947).

universe has made man as perfectly as he could make him, and he could not have invented a better device for his maintenance than to provide him with a sense of pain."[52] Leibnitz's comment on this sentence is instructive. He says first that in principle it would have been even better if God had used positive rather than negative reinforcement, inspiring pleasure each time a man turned away from the fire that could destroy him. However, he concludes that God could have succeeded with this strategy only by working miracles, and since, as a matter of principle, God avoids miracles, "pain is a necessary and brilliant device to ensure man's functioning." Within two generations of Descartes's attempt at a scientific anthropology, pain has become useful. From being the experience of the precariousness of existence,[53] it had turned into an indicator of specific breakdown.

By the end of the last century, pain had become a regulator of body functions, subject to the laws of nature; it needed no more metaphysical explanation.[54] It had ceased to deserve any mystical respect and could be subjected to empirical study in order to do away with it. By 1853, barely a century and a half after pain was recognized as a mere physiological

---

[52]Gottfried Wilhelm Leibnitz, *Essais de Théodicée sur la bonté de Dieu, la liberté de l'homme et l'origine du mal* (Paris: Garnier-Flammarion, 1969), no. 342.

[53]Pain came to be considered mysterious and unmanageable without technical aids. For orientation on the romantic attitude towards pain and the use of narcotics, see Alethea Hayter, *Opium and the Romantic Imagination* (Berkeley: Univ. of California Press, 1969). Also M. H. Abrams, *The Milk of Paradise* (New York: Harper & Row, 1970). Its avoidance became paramount: Robert Mauzi, *L'Idée du bonheur dans la littérature et la pensée françaises au 18ème siècle* (Paris: Colin, 1960), especially pp. 300–10 on the appearance of the conviction that pain is the only true evil.

[54]Charles Richet, "Douleur," in *Dictionnaire de physiologie* (Paris: Félix Alcan, 1902), 5:173–93. In his five-volume standard dictionary of physiology he analyzes pain as a physiological and psychological fact without considering either the possibility of its treatment or its diagnostic significance. Ultimately he comes to the conclusion that pain is supremely useful (*souverainement utile*) because it makes us turn away from danger. Every abuse is immediately followed for our punishment by pain, which is clearly superior in intensity to the pleasure that abuse produced.

safeguard, a medicine labeled as a "pain-killer" was marketed in La Crosse, Wisconsin.[55] A new sensibility had developed which was dissatisfied with the world, not because it was dreary or sinful or lacking in enlightenment or threatened by barbarians, but because it was full of suffering and pain.[56] Progress in civilization became synonymous with the reduction of the sum total of suffering. From then on, politics was taken to be an activity not so much for maximizing happiness as for minimizing pain. The result is a tendency to see pain as essentially a passive happening inflicted on helpless victims because the toolbox of the medical corporation is not being used in their favor.

In this context it now seems rational to flee pain rather than to face it, even at the cost of giving up intense aliveness. It seems reasonable to eliminate pain, even at the cost of losing independence. It seems enlightened to deny legitimacy to all nontechnical issues that pain raises, even if this means turning patients into pets.[57] With rising levels of induced insensitivity to pain, the capacity to experience the simple joys and pleasures of life has equally declined. Increasingly stronger stimuli are needed to provide people in an anesthetic society with any sense of being alive. Drugs, violence, and horror turn into increasingly powerful stimuli that can still elicit an experience of self. Widespread anesthesia increases the demand for excitation by noise, speed, violence—no matter how destructive.

This raised threshold of physiologically mediated

---

[55]Mitford M. Mathews, ed., *A Dictionary of Americanisms on Historical Principles* (Chicago: Univ. of Chicago Press, 1966): "*pain-killer.* Any one of various medicines or remedies for abolishing or relieving pain. 1853 La Crosse Democrat 7 June 2/4 Ayer's Cherry Pectoral, Perry Davis' Pain Killer. 1886 Ebbutt Emigrant Life 119. We kept a bottle of Pain-killer in the house . . . for medicinal purposes."

[56]Kenneth Minogue, *The Liberal Mind* (London: Methuen, 1963).

[57]Victor E. Frankl, *Homo patients: Versuch einer Pathodizee* (Vienna: Deutike, 1950).

experience, which is characteristic of a medicalized society, makes it extremely difficult today to recognize in the capacity for suffering a possible symptom of health. The reminder that suffering is a responsible activity is almost unbearable to consumers, for whom pleasure and dependence on industrial outputs coincide. By equating all personal participation in facing unavoidable pain with "masochism," they justify their passive life-style. Yet, while rejecting the acceptance of suffering as a form of masochism, anesthesia consumers tend to seek a sense of reality in ever stronger sensations. They tend to seek meaning for their lives and power over others by enduring undiagnosable pains and unrelievable anxieties: the hectic life of business executives, the self-punishment of the rat-race, and the intense exposure to violence and sadism in films and on television. In such a society the advocacy of a renewed style in the art of suffering that incorporates the competent use of new techniques will inevitably be misinterpreted as a sick desire for pain: as obscurantism, romanticism, dolorism, or sadism.

Ultimately, the management of pain might substitute a new kind of horror for suffering: the experience of artificial painlessness. Lifton describes the impact of mass death on survivors by studying people who had been close to ground zero in Hiroshima.[58] He found that people moving amongst the injured and dying simply ceased to feel; they were in a state of numbness, without emotional response. He believed that after a while this emotional closure merged with a depression which, twenty years after the bomb, still manifested itself in the guilt or shame of having survived without experiencing any pain at the time of the explosion. These people live in an interminable encounter with death which has spared them, and they suffer from a vast breakdown of trust in the larger human matrix that supports each individual human life. They experienced their anesthetized pas-

---

[58]Robert J. Lifton, *Death in Life: Survivors of Hiroshima* (New York: Random House, 1969).

sage through this event as something just as monstrous as the death of those around them, as a pain too dark and too overwhelming to be confronted, or suffered.[59]

What the bomb did in Hiroshima might guide us to an understanding of the cumulative effect on a society in which pain has been medically "expropriated." Pain loses its referential character if it is dulled, and generates a meaningless, questionless residual horror. The sufferings for which traditional cultures have evolved endurance sometimes generated unbearable anguish, tortured imprecations, and maddening blasphemies; they were also self-limiting. The new experience that has replaced dignified suffering is artificially prolonged, opaque, depersonalized maintenance. Increasingly, pain-killing turns people into unfeeling spectators of their own decaying selves.

---

[59]Terrence Des Pres, "Survivors and the Will to Bear Witness," *Social Research* 40 (winter 1973): 668–90, gives a constructive critique of Robert Lifton. According to him, the survivors of concentration camps have the urge to render significant a nameless experience they have known: pain which is utterly senseless. According to Des Pres their message is deeply offensive because since the middle of the 19th century the suffering of others has become charged with moral status. Kierkegaard preached salvation through pain, Nietzsche celebrated the abyss, Marx the downtrodden and oppressed. The survivor excites envy of his suffering, and simultaneously testifies that pain can be valued only by the privileged few.

4

The Invention and Elimination of Disease

The French Revolution gave birth to two great myths: one, that physicians could replace the clergy; the other, that with political change society would return to a state of original health.[1] Sickness became a public affair. In the name of progress, it has now ceased to be the concern of those who are ill.[2]

For several months in 1792, the National Assembly in Paris tried to decide how to replace those physicians who profited from care of the sick with a therapeutic bureaucracy designed to manage an evil that was destined to disappear with the advent of equality, freedom, and fraternity. The new priesthood was to be financed by funds expropriated from the Church. It was to guide the nation in a militant

---

[1]In this chapter I quote freely from documents gathered in Michel Foucault, *The Birth of the Clinic: An Archaeology of Medical Perception*, trans. A. M. Sheridan Smith (New York: Pantheon, 1973).

[2]Walter Artelt, *Einführung in die Medizinhistorik: Ihr Wesen, ihre Arbeitsweise und ihre Hilfsmittel* (Stuttgart: Enke, 1949). An excellent introduction to the methodology of medical history and its tools.

conversion to healthy living which would make medical sick-care less necessary. Each family would again be able to take care of its members, and each village to provide for the sick who were without relatives. A national health service would be in charge of health care and would supervise the enactment of dietary laws and of statutes compelling citizens to use their new freedoms for frugal living and wholesome pleasures. Medical officers would supervise the compliance of the citizenry, and medical magistrates would preside over health tribunals to guard against charlatans and exploiters.

Even more radical were the proposals from a subcommittee for the elimination of beggary. In content and style they are similar to Red Guard and Black Panther manifestos demanding that control over health be returned to the people. Primary care, it was asserted, belongs only to the neighborhood. Public funds for sick-care are best used to supplement the income of the afflicted. If hospitals are needed, they should be specialized: for the aged, the incurable, the mad, or foundlings. Sickness is a symptom of political corruption and will be eliminated when the government is cleaned up.

The identification of hospitals with pestholes was current and easy to explain. They had appeared under Christian auspices in late antiquity as dormitories for travelers, vagrants, and derelicts. Physicians began to visit hospitals regularly at the time of the crusades, following the example of the Arabs.[3] During the late Middle Ages, as charitable institutions for the custody of the destitute, they became part and parcel of urban architecture.[4] Until the late eigh-

---

[3]Heinrich Schipperges, "Die arabische Medizin als Praxis und als Theorie," *Sudhoffs Archiv* 43 (1959): 317–28, provides a historiographic perspective.

[4]On the evolution of the hospital as an architectonical element in urbanization, consult a dated monument: Henry Burdett, *Hospitals and Asylums of the World: Their Origin, History, Construction, Administration . . . and Legislation,* 4 vols. (London: Churchill, 1893). Also Dieter Jetter, *Geschichte des Hospitals,* vol. 1, *Westdeutschland von den Anfängen bis 1850* (Wiesbaden: Steiner, 1966); several volumes planned.

teenth century the trip to the hospital was taken, typically, with no hope of return.[5] Nobody went to a hospital to restore his health. The sick, the mad, the crippled, epileptics, incurables, foundlings, and recent amputees of all ages and both sexes were jumbled together;[6] amputations were performed in the corridors between the beds. Inmates were given some food, chaplains and pious lay folk came to offer consolation, and doctors made charity visits. The cost of remedies made up less than 3 percent of the meager budget. More than half went for the hospital soup; the nuns could get along on a pittance. Like prisons, hospitals were considered a last resort;[7] nobody thought of them as tools for administering therapy to improve the inmates.[8]

Logically, some extremists went beyond the recommendations made by the committee on beggary.

---

[5]Fernando da Silva Coreia, *Origenes e formaçaõ das misericórdias portuguesas* (Lisbon: Torres, 1944). The first two hundred pages deal with the hospital in antiquity and during the Middle Ages in the Orient and in Europe. Jean Imbert, *Histoire des hôpitaux français; contribution à l'étude des rapports de l'église et de l'état dans le domaine de l'assistance publique: les hôpitaux en droit canonique,* Collection L'Église et l'état au moyen âge, no. 8 (Paris: Vrin, 1947). Well-documented guide to the sources of the medieval hospital and the transition of public assistance from ecclesiastic to civilian control. F. N. L. Poynter, ed., *The Evolution of Hospitals in Britain* (London: Pitman, 1964); see the classified bibliography of British hospital history, pp. 255–79. For the hospital in the New World consult Josefina Muriel de la Torre, *Hospitales de la Nueva España* (vol. 1), *Fundaciones de los siglos XVII y XVIII* (vol. 2), publications of the Instituto de Historia, Universidad Nacional, ser. 1, nos. 35, 62 (Mexico, 1956–60).

[6]On the history of the hospital bed, consult F. Boinet, *Le Lit d'hôpital en France: Étude historique* (Paris: Foulton, 1945); James N. Blyth, *Notes on Beds and Bedding: Historical and Annotated* (London: Simpkin Marstall, 1873). More general, but also more pleasant reading: Laurence Wright, *Warm and Snug: The History of the Bed* (London: Routledge, 1962). On good behavior when in bed, see work by Norbert Elias cited in note 28, p. 163 below.

[7]Marcel Fosseyeux, *L'Hôtel Dieu aux XVIIe et XVIIIe siècles* (Paris: Levrault, 1912).

[8]For the origins and the evolution of the idea: David Rothman, *The Discovery of the Asylum* (Boston: Little, Brown, 1971). Milton Kotler, *Neighborhood Government: The Local Foundations of Political Life* (Indianapolis: Bobbs-Merrill, 1969), makes a clear case for Boston. See also Foucault, *Birth of the Clinic.*

Some demanded the outright abolition of all hospitals, saying that they "are inevitably places for the aggregation of the sick and breed misery while they stigmatize the patient. If a society continues to need hospitals, this is a sign that its revolution has failed."[9]

A misunderstanding of Rousseau vibrates in this desire to restore sickness to its "natural state,"[10] to bring society back to "wild sickness," which is self-limiting and can be borne with virtue and style and cared for in the homes of the poor, just as previously the sicknesses of the rich had been taken care of. Sickness becomes complex, untreatable, and unbearable only when exploitation breaks up the family,[11] and it becomes malignant and demeaning only with the advent of urbanization and civilization. For Rousseau's followers the sickness seen in hospitals was man-made, like all forms of social injustice, and it thrived among the self-indulgent and those whom they had impoverished. "In the hospital, sickness is totally corrupted; it turns into 'prison fever' characterized by spasms, fever, indigestion, pale urine, depressed respiration, and ultimately leads to death: if not on the eighth or eleventh day, then on the thirteenth."[12] It is this kind of language that made medicine first become a political issue. The plans to engineer a society into health began with the call for a social reconstruction that would eliminate the ills of civilization.

---

[9]It was enjoined on Christian princes not to use life imprisonment as a punishment because it was much too cruel. Prisons might be used to keep criminals until their hearing, their execution, or their judicial mutilation. Andreas Perneder, *Von Straff und Peen aller und jeder Malefitz handlungen ain kurtzer Bericht*, ed. W. Hunger (Ingolstadt, 1544).

[10]For documentation on the carefully qualified and rich thought of Rousseau on medicine, see Gerhard Rudolf, "Jean-Jacques Rousseau (1712–1778) und die Medizin," *Sudhoffs Archiv* 53 (1969): 30–67. Rousseau was probably misunderstood even more on medicine than on education.

[11]On the dream of "wild" health consult Edward Dudley and Maximillian E. Novak, eds., *The Wild Man Within: An Image in Western Thought from the Renaissance to Romanticism* (Pittsburgh: Pittsburgh Univ. Press, 1972).

[12]Jacques-René Tenon, *Mémoires sur les hôpitaux* (Paris, 1788), p. 451; cited in Foucault, *Birth of the Clinic*, p. 17.

What Dubos has called "the mirage of health" began as a political program.

In the public rhetoric of the 1790s, the idea of using biomedical interventions on people or on their environment was totally absent. Only with the Restoration was the task of eliminating sickness turned over to the medical profession. After the Congress of Vienna, hospitals proliferated and medical schools boomed.[13] So did the discovery of diseases. Illness was still primarily nontechnical. In 1770, general practice knew of little besides the plague and the pox,[14] but by 1860 even the ordinary citizen recognized the medical names of a dozen diseases. The sudden emergence of the doctor as savior and miracle worker was due not to the proven efficacy of new techniques but to the need for a magical ritual that would lend credibility to a pursuit at which a political revolution had failed. If "sickness" and "health" were to lay claim to public resources, then these concepts had to be made operational. Ailments had to be turned into objective diseases that infested mankind, could be transplanted and cultivated in the laboratory, and could be fitted into wards, records, budgets, and museums. Disease was thus accommodated to administrative management; one branch of the elite was entrusted by the dominant class with autonomy in its control and elimination. The object of medical treatment was defined by a new, though submerged, political ideology and acquired the status of an entity that existed quite separately from both doctor and patient.[15]

---

[13]Brian Abel-Smith, *The Hospitals, 1800–1948: A Study in Social Administration in England and Wales* (London: Heinemann, 1964). Carefully documented on economic and professional changes. Leonard K. Eaton, *New England Hospitals, 1790–1833* (Ann Arbor: Univ. of Michigan Press, 1957). See especially the bibliographical essay, pp. 239–46.

[14]François Millepierres, *La Vie quotidienne des médecins au temps de Molière* (Paris: Hachette, 1964). Popular but reliable; a composite picture of the day-by-day life of the physician at the time of Molière.

[15]Jean-Pierre Peter, "Malades et maladies à la fin du XVIIIe siècle," in Jean-Paul Dessaive et al., *Médecins, climat et épidémies*

We tend to forget how recently disease entities were born. In the mid-nineteenth century, a saying attributed to Hippocrates was still quoted with approval: "You can discover no weight, no form nor calculation to which to refer your judgment of health and sickness. In the medical arts there exists no certainty except in the physician's senses." Sickness was still personal suffering in the mirror of the doctor's vision.[16] The transformation of this medical portrait into a clinical entity represents an event in medicine that corresponds to the achievement of Copernicus in astronomy: man was catapulted and estranged from the center of his universe. Job became Prometheus.

The hope of bringing to medicine the elegance that Copernicus had given astronomy dates from the time of Galileo. Descartes traced the coordinates for the implementation of the project. His description effectively turned the human body into clockworks and placed a new distance, not only between soul and body, but also between the patient's complaint and the physician's eye. Within this mechanized framework, pain turned into a red light and sickness into mechanical trouble. A taxonomy of diseases became possible. As minerals and plants could be classified, so diseases could be isolated and categorized by the doctor-taxonomist. The logical frame-

---

à la fin du XVIIIe siècle (Paris: Mouton, 1972), pp. 135–70: "During the French Revolution the hospital, like the laboratory, both discovered around 1770, would play the midwife's role in the birth of these pre-existing ideas."

[16]Helmut Vogt, *Das Bild des Kranken: Die Darstellung äusserer Veränderungen durch innere Leiden und ihre Heilmassnahmen von der Renaissance bis zu unserer Zeit* (Munich: Lehmann, 1960). More than 500 reproductions of artistic representations of sick people since the Renaissance; allows a study of perception. For a medical study of ergotism in the past based on its representation in paintings, see Veit Harold Bauer, *Das Antonius Feuer in Kunst und Medizin* (Heidelberg: Springer, 1973); bibliog., pp. 118–25; afterword by Wolfgang Jacob, pp. 127–9. Painting and plastic arts provide an invaluable complement to the history of patient-doctor relations: Eugen Holländer, *Die Medizin in der klassischen Malerei*, 4th ed. (Stuttgart: Enke, 1950). Eugen Holländer, *Plastik und Medizin* (Stuttgart: Enke, 1912).

work for a new purpose in medicine had been laid. Instead of suffering man, sickness was placed in the center of the medical system and could be subjected to (*a*) operational verification by measurement, (*b*) clinical study and experiment, and (*c*) evaluation according to engineering norms.

Antiquity knew no yardstick for disease.[17] Galileo's contemporaries were the first to try to apply measurement to the sick, but with little success. Since Galen had taught that urine was secreted directly from the vena cava and that its composition was a direct indication of the nature of the blood, doctors had tasted and smelled urine and assayed it by the light of sun and moon. After the sixteenth century, alchemicsts had learned to measure specific gravity with considerable precision, and they subjected the urine of the sick to their methods. Dozens of distinct and differing meanings were ascribed to changes in the specific gravity of urine. With this first measurement, doctors began to read diagnostic and curative meaning into any new measurement they learned to perform.[18]

The use of physical measurements prepared for

---

[17]W. Muri, "Der Massgedanke bei griechischen Ärzten," *Gymnasium* 57 (1950): 183–201. H. Laue, *Mass und Mitte: Eine problemgeschichtliche Untersuchung zur fruehen griechischen Philosophie und Ethik* (Münster: Osnabrueck, 1960). Measure in antiquity was related to virtue and proportion, not to operational verification. On the prehistoric Indo-Germanic semantic field which includes both measure and medicine see Emile Benveniste, "Médecine et la notion de mesure," in *Le Vocabulaire des institutions indo-europêenes*, vol. 2, *Pouvoir, droit, religion*, 1969, pp. 123–32. The English version is *Indo-European Language and Society* (Miami: University of Miami Press, 1973).

[18]For the history of measurements consult two symposia: Harry Woolf, ed., *Quantification: A History of the Meaning of Measurement in the Natural and Social Sciences* (Indianapolis: Bobbs-Merrill, 1961), and Daniel Lerner, *Quantity and Quality: The Hayden Colloquium on Scientific Method and Concept* (New York: Free Press, 1961). Particularly consult, in Woolf, the paper by Richard Shryock, "The History of Quantification in Medical Science," pp. 85–107. For the application of measurement to nonmedical aspects of man, see S. S. Stevens, "Measurement and Man," *Science* 127 (1958): 383–9, and S. S. Stevens, *Handbook of Experimental Psychology* (New York: Wiley, 1951).

a belief in the real existence of diseases and their ontological autonomy from the perception of doctor and patient. The use of statistics underpinned this belief. It "showed" that diseases were present in the environment and could invade and infect people. The first clinical tests using statistics, which were performed in the United States in 1721 and published in London in 1722, provided hard data indicating that smallpox was threatening Massachusetts and that people who had been inoculated were protected against its attacks. They were conducted by Dr. Cotton Mather, who is better known for his inquisitorial fury at the time of the Salem witch trials than for his spirited defense of smallpox prevention.[19]

During the seventeenth and eighteenth centuries, doctors who applied measurements to sick people were liable to be considered quacks by their colleagues. During the French Revolution, English doctors still looked askance at clinical thermometry. Together with the routine taking of the pulse, it became accepted clinical practice only around 1845, nearly thirty years after the stethoscope was first used by Laënnec.

As the doctor's interest shifted from the sick to sickness, the hospital became a museum of disease. The wards were full of indigent people who offered their bodies as exhibits to any physician willing to treat them.[20] The realization that the hospital was the logical place to study and compare "cases" de-

---

[19]Richard H. Shryock and Otho T. Beall, *Cotton Mather: The First Significant Figure in American Medicine* (Baltimore: Johns Hopkins Univ. Press, 1954).

[20]When disease became an entity that could be separated from man and dealt with by the doctor, other aspects of man suddenly became detachable, usable, salable. The sale of the shadow is a typically 19th-century literary motif (A. V. Chamisso, *Peter Schlemihls wundersame Geschichte,* 1814). A demoniacal doctor can deprive man of his mirror-image (E. T. A. Hoffman, "Die Geschichte vom verlorenen Spiegelbild," in *Die Abenteuer einer Sylvesnacht,* 1815). In W. Hauff, "Des steinerne Hertz," in *Das Wirtshaus im Spessat* (1828), the hero exchanges his heart for one of stone to save himself from bankruptcy. Within the next two generations, literary treatment was given to the sale of appetite, name, youth, and memories.

veloped towards the end of the eighteenth century. Doctors visited hospitals where all kinds of sick people were mingled, and trained themselves to pick out several "cases" of the same disease. They developed "bedside vision," or a clinical eye. During the first decades of the nineteenth century, the medical attitude towards hospitals went through a further development. Until then, new doctors had been trained mostly by lectures, demonstrations, and disputations. Now the "bedside" became the clinic, the place where future doctors were trained to see and recognize diseases.[21] The clinical approach to sickness gave birth to a new language which spoke about diseases at the bedside, and to a hospital reorganized and classified by disease for the exhibition of ailments to students.[22]

The hospital, which at the very beginning of the nineteenth century had become a place for diagnosis, was now turned into a place for teaching. Soon it would become a laboratory for experimenting with treatments, and towards the turn of the century a place concerned with therapy. Today the pesthouse has been transformed into a compartmentalized repair shop. All this happened in stages. During the nineteenth century, the clinic became the place where disease carriers were assembled, diseases were identified, and a census of diseases was kept. Medical perception of reality became hospital-based much

---

[21]For this evolution in France, see Maurice Rochaix, *Essai sur l'évolution des questions hospitalières de la fin de l'Ancien Régime à nos jours* (Saintes: Fédération hospitalière de France, 1959), the only well-documented history of public assistance to the sick in France. See Jean Imbert, *Les Hôpitaux en France*, "Que sais-je?" (Paris: Presses Universitaires de France, 1958), on the adaptation of the French hospital to changing medical techniques during the 19th century. Of course, consult also Foucault, *Birth of the Clinic.*

[22]On the history of the concept of disease, see P. Diepgen, G. B. Gruber, and H. Schadewaldt, "Der Krankheitsbegriff, seine Geschichte und Problematik," in *Prologomena einer allgemeinen Pathologie* (Berlin: Springer, 1969), 1:1–50. Emanuel Berghoff, *Entwicklungsgeschichte des Krankheitsbegriffes: In seinen Hauptzügen dargestellt*, 2nd ed., Wiener Beiträge zur Geschichte der Medizin, vol. 1 (Vienna: Maudrich, 1947). Pedro Lain Entralgo, *El médico y el enfermo* (Madrid: Ediciones Guadarrama, 1970).

earlier than medical practice. The specialized hospital demanded by the French Revolutionaries for the sake of the patient became a reality because doctors needed to classify sickness. During the entire nineteenth century, pathology remained overwhelmingly the classification of anatomical anomalies. Only towards the end of the century did the pupils of Claude Bernard also begin to label and catalogue the pathology of functions.[23] Like sickness, health acquired a clinical status, becoming the absence of clinical symptoms, and clinical standards of normality became associated with well-being.[24]

Disease could never have been associated with abnormality if the value of universal standards had not come to be recognized in one field after another over a period of two hundred years. In 1635, at the behest of Cardinal Richelieu, the king of France formed an academy of the forty supposedly most distinguished men of French letters for the purpose of protecting and perfecting the French language. In fact, they imposed the language of the rising bourgeoisie which was also gaining control over the expanding tools of production. The language of the new class of capitalist producers became normative for all classes. State authority had expanded beyond statute law to regulate means of expression. Citizens learned to recognize the normative power of an elite in areas left untouched by the canons of the Church and the civil and penal codes of the state. Offenses against the codified laws of French grammar now carried their own sanctions; they put the speaker in his place —that is, deprived him of the privileges of class

---

[23]Mirko D. Grmek, "La Conception de la maladie et de la santé chez Claude Bernard," in Alexandre Koyré, *Mélanges Alexandre Koyré: L'Aventure de la science* (Paris: Hermann, 1964), 1:208–27.

[24]Georges Canguilhem, *Le Normal et le pathologique* (Paris: Presses Universitaires de France, 1972), is a thesis on the history of the idea of normalcy in 19th-century pathology, finished in 1943 with a postscript in 1966. On the history of "normality" in psychiatry see Michel Foucault, *Madness and Civilization: A History of Insanity in the Age of Reason* (New York: Pantheon, 1965).

and profession. Bad French was that which fell below academic standards, as bad health would soon be that which was not up to the clinical norm.

In Latin *norma* means "square," the carpenter's square. Until the 1830s the English word "normal" meant standing at a right angle to the ground. During the 1840s it came to designate conformity to a common type. In the 1880s, in America, it came to mean the usual state or condition not only of things but also of people. In France, the word was transposed from geometry to society—*école normale* designated a school at which teachers for the Empire were trained—and was first given a medical connotation around 1840 by Auguste Comte. He expressed his hope that once the laws relative to the normal state of the organism were known, it would be possible to engage in the study of comparative pathology.[25]

During the last decade of the nineteenth century, the norms and standards of the hospital became fundamental criteria for diagnosis and therapy. For this to happen, it was not necessary that all abnormal features be considered pathological; it was sufficient that disease as deviance from a clinical standard make

[25]For the history of medical ideas during the 19th century, see Pedro Lain Entralgo, *La medicina hipocrática* (Madrid: Revista de Occidente, 1970). Werner Leibrand, *Heilkunde: Eine Problemsgeschichte der Medizin* (Freiburg: Alber, 1953). Fritz Hartmann, *Der ärztliche Auftrag: Die Entwicklung der Idee des abendländischen Arzttums aus ihren weltanschaulich-anthropologischen Voraussetzungen bis zum Beginn der Neuzeit* (Göttingen: Musterschmidt, 1956). M. Merleau-Ponty, "L'Oeil de l'esprit," *Les Temps Modernes*, nos. 184–5 (1961), pp. 193 ff. M. Merleau-Ponty, *Phénoménologie de la perception* (Paris: Gallimard, 1945). Werner Leibrand, *Spekulative Medizin der Romantik* (Hamburg: Claassen, 1956). Hans Freyer, "Der Arzt und die Gesellschaft," in *Der Arzt und der Staat* (Leipzig: Thieme 1929). René Fülop-Miller, *Kulturgeschichte der Heilkunde* (Munich: Bruckmann, 1937). K. E. Hrag Rothschuh, *Was ist Krankheit? Erscheinung, Erklärung, Sinngebung*, Wege der Forschung, vol. 362 (Darmstadt: Wissenschaftliche Buchgesellschaft, 1976): 18 historically important critical contributions of the 19th and 20th centuries to the epistemology of sickness, among them C. W. Hufeland, R. Virchow, R. Koch, and F. Alexander. Richard Toellner will publish a parallel volume, *Erfahrung und Denken in der Medizin*.

medical intervention legitimate by providing an orientation for therapy.[26]

The age of hospital medicine, which from rise to fall lasted no more than a century and a half, is coming to an end.[27] Clinical measurement has been diffused throughout society. Society has become a clinic, and all citizens have become patients whose blood pressure is constantly being watched and regulated to fall "within" normal limits. The acute problems of manpower, money, access, and control that beset hospitals everywhere can be interpreted as symptoms of a new crisis in the concept of disease. This is a true crisis because it admits of two opposing solutions, both of which make present hospitals obsolete. The first solution is a further sickening medicalization of health care, expanding still further the clinical control of the medical profession over the ambulatory population. The second is a critical, scientifically sound demedicalization of the concept of disease.

Medical epistemology is much more important for the healthy solution of this crisis than either medical biology or medical technology. Such an epistemology will have to clarify the logical status and the social nature of diagnosis and therapy, primarily in physical—as opposed to mental—sickness. All disease is a socially created reality. Its meaning and

---

[26]On this development, especially as it centered around the influence of Virchow, see Wolfgang Jacob, "Medizinische Anthropologie im 19. Jh.: Mensch, Natur, Gesellschaft: Beitrag zu einer theoretischen Pathologie," in *Beiträge aus der allgemeinen Medizin,* no. 20 (Stuttgart: Enke, 1967).

[27]Janine Ferry-Pierret and Serge Karsenty, *Pratiques médicales et système hospitalier* (Paris: CEREBE, 1974), an economic analysis of the rising marginal disutilities to health care which have resulted from a take-over by the hospital in medical care (the takeover was possible because of a hospital-centered perception of disease). For a dozen sociological perspectives on the contemporary hospital, consult Eliot Freidson, ed., *The Hospital in Modern Society* (New York: Free Press, 1963). See also Johann J. Rhode, *Soziologie des Krankenhauses: Zur Einführung in die Soziologie der Medizin . . .* (Stuttgart: Enke, 1962), perhaps the most comprehensive sociology of the hospital.

the response it has evoked have a history.[28] The study of this history will make us understand the degree to which we are prisoners of the medical ideology in which we were brought up.

A number of authors have recently tried to debunk the status of *mental* deviance as a "disease."[29] Paradoxically, they have rendered it more and not less difficult to raise the same kind of question about *disease in general.* Leifer, Goffman, Szasz, Laing, and others are all interested in the political genesis of mental illness and its use for political purposes.[30] In order to make their point, they all contrast "unreal" mental with "real" physical disease: in their view the language of natural science, now applied to all conditions that are studied by physicians, really fits physical sickness only. Physical sickness is confined to the body, and it lies in an anatomical, physiological, and genetic context. The "real" existence of these conditions can be confirmed by measurement and experiment, without any reference to a value-system. None of this applies to mental sickness: its status as

---

[28]On the history of body perception in European cultures, see Norbert Elias, *Über den Prozess der Zivilisation: Soziogenetische und psychogenetische Untersuchungen,* vol. 1, *Wandlungen des Verhaltens in den Weltlichten des Abendlandes;* vol. 2, *Wandlungen der Gesellschaft Entwurf zu einer Theorie der Zivilisation* (Bern/Munich: Francke, 1969). (French translation, Paris: Calmann-Levy, 1973).

[29]An example: D. L. Rosenhan, "On Being Sane in Insane Places," *Science* 179 (1973): 250–58. "Once eight pseudopatients had gained admission to mental institutions (by saying they heard voices), they found themselves indelibly labeled with a diagnosis of schizophrenia—in spite of their subsequent normal behavior. Ironically, it was only the other inmates who suspected that the pseudopatients were normal. The hospital personnel were not able to acknowledge normal behavior within the hospital milieu."

[30]Thomas S. Szasz, *The Myth of Mental Illness* (New York: Harper & Row, 1961). Thomas S. Szasz, *Manufacture of Madness: A Comparative Study of the Inquisition and the Mental Health Movement* (New York: Harper & Row, 1970). Ronald Leifer, *In the Name of Mental Health: Social Functions of Psychiatry* (New York: Aronson, 1969). Erving Goffman, *Asylums: Essays on the Social Situation of Mental Patients and Other Inmates* (1961; paperback ed., New York: Doubleday, 1973). R. D. Laing and A. Esterson, *Sanity, Madness, and the Family* (Baltimore: Penguin, 1970).

a "sickness" depends entirely on psychiatric judgment. The psychiatrist acts as the agent of a social, ethical, and political milieu. Measurements and experiments on these "mental" conditions can be conducted only within an ideological framework which derives its consistency from the general social prejudice of the psychiatrist. The prevalence of sickness is blamed on life in an alienated society, but while political reconstruction might eliminate much psychic sickness, it would merely provide better and more equitable technical treatment for those who are physically ill.

This antipsychiatric stance, which legitimizes the nonpolitical status of physical disease by denying to mental deviance the character of disease, is a minority position in the West, although it seems to be close to an official doctrine in modern China, where mental illness is perceived as a political problem. Maoist politicians are placed in charge of psychotic deviants. Bermann[31] reports that the Chinese object to the revisionist Russian practice of depoliticizing the deviance of class enemies by locking them into hospitals and treating them as if they had a sickness and analogous to an infection. They pretend that only the opposite approach can give results: the intensive political re-education of people who are now, perhaps unconsciously, class enemies. Their self-criticism will make them politically active and thus healthy. Here again, the insistence on the primarily nonclinical nature of mental deviance reinforces the belief that another kind of sickness is a material entity.[32]

Advanced industrial societies have a high stake in maintaining the epistemological legitimacy of dis-

---

[31] Gregoria Bermann, *La Santé mentale en Chine,* trans. A. Barbaste (Paris: Maspero, 1974). Original title: *La salud mental en China* (Buenos Aires: Ed. Jorge Alvarez, 1970).

[32] Peter Sedgwick, "Illness, Mental and Otherwise: All Illnesses Express a Social Judgement," *Hastings Center Studies* 1, no. 3 (1973): 19–40, points out that events constitute sickness and disease only after man labels them both as deviances and as conditions that are under social control. He promises to raise the epistomological question about sickness in general in a book soon to be published by Harper & Row.

ease entities. As long as disease is something that takes possession of people, something they "catch" or "get," the victims of these natural processes can be exempted from responsibility for their condition. They can be pitied rather than blamed for sloppy, vile, or incompetent performance in suffering their subjective reality; they can be turned into manageable and profitable assets if they humbly accept their disease as the expression of "how things are"; and they can be discharged from any political responsibility for having collaborated in increasing the sickening stress of high-intensity industry. An advanced industrial society is sick-making because it disables people to cope with their environment and, when they break down, it substitutes a "clinical" prosthesis for the broken *relationships*. People would rebel against such an environment if medicine did not explain their biological disorientation as a defect in their health, rather than as a defect in the way of life which is imposed on them or which they impose on themselves.[33] The assurance of personal political innocence that a diagnosis offers the patient serves as a hygienic mask that justifies further subjection to production and consumption.

The medical diagnosis of substantive disease entities that supposedly take shape in the individual's body is a surreptitious and amoral way of blaming the victim. The physician, himself a member of the dominating class, judges that the individual does not fit into an environment that has been engineered and is administered by other professionals, instead of accusing his colleagues of creating environments into which the human organism cannot fit. Substantive disease can thus be interpreted as the materialization of a politically convenient myth, which takes on substance within the individual's body when this body is in rebellion against the demands that industrial society makes upon it.

---

[33]Albert Görres, "Sinn und Unsinn der Krankheit: Hiob und Freud," in Albert Görres, ed., *Der Kranke, Ärgernis der Leistungsgesellschaft* (Düsseldorf: Patmos, 1971), pp. 74–88.

In every society the classification of disease—the nosology—mirrors social organization. The sickness that society produces is baptized by the doctor with names that bureaucrats cherish. "Learning disability," "hyperkinesis," or "minimal brain dysfunction" explains to parents why their children do not learn, serving as an alibi for the school's intolerance or incompetence; high blood pressure serves as an alibi for mounting stress, degenerative disease for degenerating social organization. The more convincing the diagnosis, the more valuable the therapy appears to be, the easier it is to convince people that they need both, and the less likely they are to rebel against industrial growth. Unionized workers demand the most costly therapy possible, if for no other reason than for the perverse pleasure of getting back some of the money they have put into taxes and insurance, and deluding themselves that this will create more equality.

Before sickness came to be perceived primarily as an organic or behavioral abnormality, he who got sick could still find in the eyes of the doctor a reflection of his own anguish and some recognition of the uniqueness of his suffering. Now, what he meets is the gaze of a biological accountant engaged in input/output calculations. His sickness is taken from him and turned into the raw material for an institutional enterprise. His condition is interpreted according to a set of abstract rules in a language he cannot understand. He is taught about alien entities that the doctor combats, but only just as much as the doctor considers necessary to gain the patient's cooperation. Language is taken over by the doctors: the sick person is deprived of meaningful words for his anguish, which is thus further increased by linguistic mystification.[34]

---

[34]B. L. Whorf, *Language, Thought and Reality* (New York: Wiley, 1956), describes the language barrier that technical terminology creates between the professional ingroup and the clients defined as the outgroup. K. Engelhardt et al., *Kranke im Krankenhaus* (Stuttgart: Enke, 1973). While at the hospital, patients are intensively and progressively mystified. At the time of dismissal less than one-third

Before scientific slang had come to dominate language about the body, the repertory of ordinary speech in this field was exceptionally rich.[35] Peasant language preserved much of this treasure into our century.[36] Proverbs and sayings kept instructions readily available.[37] The way complaints to the doctor were formulated by Babylonians and Greeks has been compared with the expressions used by German blue-collar workers. As in antiquity the patient stutters, flounders, and speaks about what "grips him" or what he "has caught." But while the industrial worker refers to his ache as a drab "it" that hurts, his predecessors had many colorful and expressive names for the demons[38] that bit or stung them. Finally, increasing dependence of socially acceptable speech on the special language of an elite profession makes

---

have understood what disease they have been treated for, and less than one-fourth, what therapy they have been subjected to. M. B. Korsch and V. F. Negrete, "Doctor-Patient Communication," *Scientific American* 227 (August 1972): 66–9. In Los Angeles Childrens' Hospital, 20% of mothers do not understand what ails their children, 50% do not grasp the origins of their disease, and 42% do not follow the advice they receive, frequently because they cannot grasp it. Raoul Carson, in *Les Vieilles Douleurs,* rev. ed. (Paris: Julliard, 1960), confirms in a more intuitive fashion that the same is true for his French patients.

[35]For the language of disease in Mediterranean antiquity see Nadia van Brock, *Recherches sur le vocabulaire médical du Grec ancien: Soins et guérison* (Paris: Klincksieck, 1961). Hermann Grapow, *Kranker, Krankheiten und Arzt: Vom gesunden und kranken Ägypter, von den Krankheiten, vom Arzt und von der ärztlichen Tätigkeit* (Berlin: Akademie-Verlag, 1956), 7:168. Georges Contenau, *La Médicine en Assyrie et en Babylonie* (Paris: Librairie Maloine, 1938). For the language of the Bible on disease, see references of note 44, p. 144 above.

[36]Max Höfler, *Deutsches Krankheitsnamen-Buch* (Munich: Piloty & Löhle, 1899). A monumental collection of German popular expressions relating to organs, their functions, and disease in man and domestic animals, as well as those which designate remedies, natural or magical; 922 packed pages.

[37]Otto E. Moll, *Sprichwörter—Bibliographie* (Frankfurt am Main: Klostermann, 1958), lists 58 collections of proverbs in all languages dealing with "health, sickness, medicine, hygiene, stupidity, and laziness" (pp. 534–7). In contrast, for a history of medical language see Johannes Steudel, *Die Sprache des Arztes: Ethymologie und Geschichte medizinischer Termini* (seen only in extracts).

[38]Dietlinde Goltz, "Krankheit und Sprache," *Sudhoffs* Archiv 53, no. 3 (1969): 225–69.

disease into an instrument of class domination. The university-trained and the bureaucrat thus become their doctor's colleague in the treatment he dispenses, while the worker is put in his place as a subject who does not speak the language of his master.[39]

As soon as medical effectiveness is assessed in ordinary language, it immediately appears that most effective diagnosis and treatment do not go beyond the understanding that any layman can develop. In fact, the overwhelming majority of diagnostic and therapeutic interventions that demonstrably do more good than harm have two characteristics: the material resources for them are extremely cheap, and they can be packaged and designed for self-use or application by family members. For example, the price of what is significantly health-furthering in Canadian medicine is so low that these same resources

---

[39]During the 19th century the new middle classes developed a sense of guilt or shame about disease, while the upper bourgeoisie and nobility turned their need for constant health care into an excuse for fashionable "cures," particularly at spas. The "season" at the great spas played a political function analogous to summit meetings today. See Walter Rüegg, "Der Kranke in der Sicht der bürgerlichen Gesellschaft an der Schwelle des 19. Jahrhunderts," and Johannes Steudel, "Therapeutische und soziologische Funktion der Mineralbäder im 19. Jahrhundert," both in Walter Artelt and Walter Rüegg, eds., *Der Arzt und der Kranke in der Gesellschaft des 19. Jahrhunderts: Vorträge eines Symposions vom 1.–3. April, 1963 in Frankfurt a.M.*, Studien zur Medizingeschichte des 19. Jahrhunderts, vol. 1 (Stuttgart: Enke, 1967). R. H. Shryock, "Medicine and Society in the 19th Century," *Cahiers d'histoire mondiale* 5 (1959): 116–46. Luc Boltanski, "La Découverte de la maladie: La Diffusion du savoir médical," mimeographed, Centre de Sociologie Européenne (Paris, 1968). Based on much empirical data, this paper gathers evidence for the class-specific diffusion of medical civilization, and shows the economic origin of the poor man's "hardiness" in the face of suffering and contrasts it with the middle-class "struggle against pain."

One way to explore reactions against the medicalization of disease perception is to study the history of humor whose butt is the doctor. Materials on caricatures can be found in U.S. National Library of Medicine, *Caricatures from the Art Collection*, comp. Sheila Durling (Washington, D.C., 1959); Helmut Vogt, *Medizinische Karikaturen von 1800 bis zur Gegenwart* (Munich: Lehmann, 1960); Curt Proskauer and Fritz Witt, *Pictorial History of Dentistry* (Cologne: Dumont, 1970); A. Weber, *Tableau de la caricature médicale depuis les origines jusqu'à nos jours* (Paris: Editions Hippocrate, 1936).

could be made available to the entire population of India for the amount of money now squandered there on modern medicine. The skills needed for the application of the most generally used diagnostic and therapeutic aids are so elementary that the careful following of instructions by people who are personally concerned would probaby guarantee more effective and responsible use than medical practice ever could. Most of what remains could probably be handled better by "barefoot" nonprofessional amateurs with deep personal commitment than by professional physicians, psychiatrists, dentists, midwives, physiotherapists, or oculists.

When the evidence about the simplicity of effective modern medicine is discussed, medicalized people usually object by saying that sick people are anxious and emotionally incompetent for rational self-medication, and that even doctors call in a colleague to treat their own sick child; and furthermore, that malevolent amateurs could quickly organize into monopoly custodians of scarce and precious medical knowledge. These objections are all valid if raised within a society in which consumer expectations shape attitudes to service, in which medical resources are carefully packaged for hospital use, and in which the mythology of medical efficiency prevails. They would hardly be valid in a world that aimed at the effective pursuit of personal goals that an austere use of technology had put within the range of almost everyone.

5

Death Against Death

Death as Commodity

In every society the dominant image of death determines the prevalent concept of health.[1] Such an image, the culturally conditioned anticipation of a

---

[1]Robert G. Olson, "Death," in *Encyclopedia of Philosophy,* ed. P. Edwards (New York: Macmillan, 1967), 2:307–9, gives a short and lucid introduction to the knowledge of death and of the fear of death. Herman Feifel, ed., *The Meaning of Death* (New York: McGraw-Hill, 1959), gave a major impetus to the psychological research on death in the U.S. Robert Fulton, ed., *Death and Identity* (New York: Wiley, 1965), is an outstanding anthology of short contributions which together reflect the stage of English-language research in 1965. Paul Landsberg, *Essai sur l'expérience de la mort, suivi de Problème moral de suicide* (Paris: Seuil, 1951), is a classic analysis. José Echeverría, *Réflexions métaphysiques sur la mort et le problème du sujet* (Paris: J. Vrin, 1957), is a lucid attempt at a phenomenology of death. Christian von Ferber, "Soziologische Aspekte des Todes: Ein Versuch über einige Beziehungen der Soziologie zur philosophischen Anthropologie," *Zeitschrift für evangelische Ethnik* 7 (1963): 338–60. A strong argument to render death again a serious public problem. The author believes that death repressed, rendered private and a matter for professionals only, reinforces the exploitative class structure of society. A very important article. See also Vladimir Jankelevitch, *La mort* (Paris: Flammarion, 1966), and Edgar Morin, *L'Homme et la mort* (Paris: Seuil, 1970).

certain event at an uncertain date, is shaped by institutional structures, deep-seated myths, and the social character that predominates. A society's image of death reveals the level of independence of its people, their personal relatedness, self-reliance, and aliveness.[2] Wherever the metropolitan medical civilization has penetrated, a novel image of death has been imported. Insofar as this image depends on the new techniques and their corresponding ethos, it is supranational in character. But these very techniques are not culturally neutral; they assumed concrete shape within Western cultures and express a Western ethos. The white man's image of death has spread with medical civilization and has been a major force in cultural colonization.

The image of a "natural death," a death which comes under medical care and finds us in good health and old age, is a quite recent ideal.[3] In five

---

[2]For the study of the antique death-image in our general context, the following are useful: Fielding H. Garrison, "The Greek Cult of the Dead and the Chthonian Deities in Ancient Medicine," *Annals of Medical History* 1 (1917): 35–53. Alice Walton, *The Cult of Asklepios,* Cornell Studies in Classical Philology no. 3 (1894; reprint ed., New York: Johnson Reprint Corp., 1965). Ernst Benz, *Das Todesproblem in der stoischen Philosophie* (Stuttgart: Kohlhammer, 1929), XI, Tübinger Beiträge zur Altertumswiss. 7. Ludwig Wachter, *Der Tod im alten Testament* (Stuttgart: Calwer, 1967). Jocelyn Mary Catherine Toynbee, *Death and Burial in the Roman World* (London: Thames & Hudson, 1971). K. Sauer, *Untersuchungen zur Darstellung des Todes in der griechisch-römischen Geschichtsschreibung* (Frankfurt, 1930). J. Kroll, "Tod und Teufel in der Antike," *Verhandlungen der Versammlung deutscher Philologen* 56 (1926). Hugo Blummer, "Die Schilderung des Sterbens in der griechischen Dichtkunst," *Neue Jahrbücher des klassischen Altertums,* 1917, pp. 499–512.

[3]This chapter leans heavily on the masterful essays by Philippe Ariés: "Le Culte des morts à l'époque moderne," *Revue de l'Académie des Sciences morales et politiques,* 1967, pp. 25–40; "La Mort inversée: Le Changement des attitudes devant la mort dans les sociétés occidentales," *Archives européennes de sociologie* 8, no. 2 (1967); "La Vie et la mort chez les français d'aujourd'hui," *Ethnopsychologie* 27 (March 1972): 39–44; "La Mort et le mourant dans notre civilisation," *Revue française de sociologie* 14 (January–March 1973); "Les Techniques de la mort," in *Histoire des populations françaises et de leurs attitudes devant la vie depuis le XVIIIe siècle* (1948; Paris: Seuil, 1971), pp. 373–98. A synopsis in English: Philippe Ariés, *Western Attitudes Towards Death: From the Middle*

hundred years it has evolved through five distinct stages, and is now ready for a sixth. Each stage has found its iconographic expression: (1) the fifteenth-century "dance of the dead"; (2) the Renaissance dance at the bidding of the skeleton man, the so-called "Dance of Death"; (3) the bedroom scene of the aging lecher under the Ancien Régime; (4) the nineteenth-century doctor in his struggle against the roaming phantoms of consumption and pestilence; (5) the mid-twentieth-century doctor who steps between the patient and his death; and (6) death under intensive hospital care. At each stage of its evolution the image of natural death has elicited a new set of responses that increasingly acquired a medical character. The history of natural death is the history of the medicalization of the struggle against death.[4]

The Devotional Dance of the Dead

From the fourth century onwards, the Church struggled against a pagan tradition in which crowds, naked, frenzied, and brandishing swords, danced on the tombs in the churchyard. Nevertheless, the frequency of ecclesiastical prohibitions testifies that they were of little avail, and for a thousand years Christian churches and cemeteries remained dance floors. Death was an occasion for the renewal of life. Danc-

---

Ages to the Present, trans. Patricia Ranum (Baltimore: Johns Hopkins, 1974; London: Marion Boyars, 1976). "La Mort inversée" appeared in a translation by Bernard Murchland as "Death Inside Out" in *Hastings Center Studies* 2 (May 1974): 3–18 (the bibliography is absent from the translation).

[4]In this chapter I am interested, above all, in the image of "natural death." I am using the term "natural death" because I find it widely used between the sixteenth and early twentieth centuries. I oppose it to "primitive death," which comes through the activities of some fey, eerie, supernatural, or divine agent, and to "contemporary death," which more often than not is conceived as a result of a social injustice, as the outcome of class struggle or of imperial domination. I am interested in the *image* of this natural death, and its evolution during the four centuries in which it was common in Western civilizations. I owe the idea of approaching my subject in this way to Werner Fuchs, *Todesbilder in der modernen Gesellschaft* (Frankfurt: Suhrkamp, 1969). On my disagreement with the author, see note 54, p. 199 below.

ing with the dead on their tombs was an occasion for affirming the joy of being alive and a source of many erotic songs and poems.[5] By the late fourteenth century, however, the sense of these dances seems to have changed:[6] from an encounter between the living and those who were already dead, it was transformed into a meditative, introspective experience. In 1424 the first Dance of the Dead was painted on a cemetery wall in Paris. The original of the Cimetière des Innocents is lost, but good copies allow us to reconstruct it: king, peasant, pope, scribe, and maiden each dance with a corpse. Each partner is a mirror image of the other in dress and feature. In the shape of his body Everyman carries his own death with him and dances with it through his life. During the late Middle Ages, indwelling death[7] faces man; each

---

[5]Thomas Ohm, *Die Gebetsgebärden der Völker und das Christentum* (Leiden: Brill, 1948), pp. 372 ff., especially pp. 389–90, collects evidence on dances held in cemeteries and the struggle of the church authorities against them. A medical history of Occidental religious choreomania: E. L. Backman, *Religious Dances in the Christian Church and in Popular Medicine* (Stockholm, 1948); trans. E. Classen (London: Allen & Unwin, 1952). A bibliography of the religious aspects of dancing: Émile Bertaud, "Danse religieuse," in *Dictionnaire de spiritualité,* fascicles 18–19, pp. 21–37. A. Schimmel, "Tanz: I. Religiongeschichtlich," in *Die Religion in Geschichte und Gegenwart* (Tübingen: 1962), 6:612–14. For the history of dances in or around Christian churches, see L. Gougaud, "La Danse dans les églises," *Revue d'histoire ecclésiastique* 15 (1914): 5–22, 229–45. J. Baloch, "Tänze in Kirche und Kirchhöfen," *Niederdeutsche Zeitschrift für Volkskunde,* 1928. H. Spanke, "Tanzmusik in der Kirche des Mittelalters," *Neuphilosophische Mitteilungen* 31 (1930). Germanic precedents to Christian cemetery dances: Richard Wolfram, *Schwerttanz und Männerbund* (Kassel: Bärenreiter, 1937); only partly in print. Werner Danckert, "Totengräber," in *Unehrliche Leute: Die verfehmten Berufe* (Bern: Francke, 1963), pp. 50–6.

[6]Johan Huizinga, "The Vision of Death," in *The Waning of the Middle Ages: A Study of the Forms of Life, Art, and Thought in France and the Netherlands in the XIVth and XVth Centuries* (New York: St. Martin, 1924), chap. 11, pp. 124–35.

[7]Gerhart B. Ladner, *The Idea of Reform: Its Impact on Christian Thought and Action in the Age of the Fathers* (Cambridge: Harvard Univ. Press, 1959). Consult p. 163 for the two currents within the Church about the relation of death to nature since the fourth century. For Pelagius death was not a punishment for sin, and Adam would have died even had he not sinned. In this he differs from Augustine's doctrine that Adam had been given immortality as a

death comes with the symbol corresponding to his victim's rank: for the king a crown, for the peasant a pitchfork. From dancing with dead ancestors over their graves, people turned to representing a world in which everyone dances through life embracing his own mortality. Death was represented, not as an anthropomorphic figure, but as a macabre self-consciousness, a constant awareness of the gaping grave. It was not yet the skeleton man of the next century to whose music men and women will soon dance through the autumn of the Middle Ages, but rather each one's own aging and rotting self.[8] At this time the mirror[9] became important in everyday life, and

---

special gift from God, and even more from those Greek Church Fathers according to whom Adam had a spiritual, or "resurrectional," body before he transgressed.

[8]So far the deceased had appeared ageless on his funeral monument. He now appears as a decaying corpse. Kathleen Cohen, *Metamorphosis of a Death Symbol: The Transi-Tomb in the Late Middle Ages and the Renaissance* (Los Angeles: Univ. of California Press, 1973). Gruesome tombs meant to teach the living appear first in the last years of the 14th century. J. P. Hornung, *Ein Beitrag zur Ikonographie des Todes,* dissertation, Univ. of Freiburg, 1902. The encounter between the living and the dead takes on importance in a new literary genre: Stefan Glixelli, *Les Cinq Poèmes des trois morts et des trois vifs* (Paris: H. Champion, 1914); J. S. Egilsrud *Le Dialogue des morts dans les littératures française, allemande et anglaise* (Paris: L'Entente linotypiste, 1934); Kaulfuss-Diesch, "Totengespräche," in *Reallexikon der deutschen Literaturgeschichte,* 3:379 ff.; and finds a new visual expression: Karl Kunstle, *Die Legende der drei Lebenden und der drei Toten* (Freiburg: Herder, 1908); Willy Rotzler, *Die Begegnung der drei Lebenden und der drei Toten: Ein Beitrag zur Forschung über mittelalterliche Vergänglichkeitsdarstellung* (Wintertur: Keller, 1961); Pierre Michault, *Pas de la mort,* ed. Jules Petit (Société des Bibliophiles de Belgique, 1869); Albert Freybe, *Das memento mori in deutscher Sitte, bildlicher Darstellung und Volksglauben, deutsche Sprache, Dichtung und Seelsorge* (Gotha: Perthes, 1909). The fact that around 1500 death assumes strong skeletal features and a new autonomy does not mean that it had not always borne anthropomorphic features, if not in art, then in legend and poetry. Paul Geiger, "Tod: 4. Der Tod als Person," in *Handwörterbuch des deutschen Aberglaubens* (Berlin: W. de Gruyter, 1927–42), 8:976–85.

[9]The one great book on the mirror in painting is G. F. Hartlaub, *Zauber des Spiegels: Geschichte und Bedeutung des Spiegels in der Kunst* (Munich: Piper, 1951). Chap. 7, sec. iii, "Spiegel der Vanitas," deals particularly with the mirror as reminder of transitoriness. See also G. F. Hartlaub, "Die Spiegel-bilder des Giovanni Bellini," *Pantheon* 15 (November 1942): 235–41. The interpretation of

in the grip of the "mirror of death" the "world"[10] acquired a hallucinating poignancy. With Chaucer and Villon, death becomes as intimate and sensual as pleasure and pain.

Primitive societies conceived of death as the result of an intervention by an alien actor. They did not attribute personality to death. Death is the outcome of someone's evil intention. This somebody who causes death might be a neighbor who, in envy, looks at you with an evil eye, or it might be a witch, an ancestor who comes to pick you up, or the black cat that crosses your path.[11] Throughout the Christian

---

Bellini's use of the mirror to depict the intensity of the new awareness of the ambiguity of human anatomy. Henrich Schwarz, "The Mirror in Art," *Art Quarterly* 15 (1952): 96–118. Specifically on "vanity."

[10]Wolfgang Stammler, *Frau Welt: Eine mittelalterliche Allegorie*, Freiburger Universitatsreden, 1959. The "world" depicted as a female figure in medieval art—half angel, half demon—represents the power of this-worldly goods, the beauty of nature, but also the decay of all that is human.

[11]For a bibliography on attitudes towards death among primitive people, see Edgar Herzog, *Psyche and Death: Archaic Myths and Modern Dreams in Analytical Psychology* (New York: Putnam, 1967). Primitive death is always conceived of as the result of intervention by an agent. For the purposes of my argument, the nature of this agent is unimportant. Though dated, Robert Hertz, "Contribution à une étude sur la représentation collective de la mort," *L'Année sociologique* 10 (1905–1906): 48–137, remains the best repository for older literature on this point. Complement with E. S. Hartland et al., "Death and the Disposal of the Dead," in *Encyclopaedia of Religion and Ethics* (1925–32), 4:411–511. Rosalind Moss, *The Life After Death in Oceania and the Malay Archipelago* (1925; Ann Arbor, Mich.: University Microfilms, 1972), shows that the burial forms tend to influence beliefs about the cause of death and the nature of the afterlife. Hans Kelsen, "Seele und Recht," in *Aufsätze zur Ideologiekritik* (Neuwied/Berlin: Luchterhand, 1964), suggests that the universal fear of murderous ancestors underpins social control. Consult also the following works by James George Frazer: *Man, God and Immortality* (London: MacMillan, 1927); *The Belief in Immortality and the Worship of the Dead*, vol. 1, *The Belief Among the Aborigines of Australia, the Torres Straits Islands, New Guinea and Melanesia* (1911: reprint ed., New York: Barnes & Noble, 1968); *The Fear of the Dead in Primitive Religion* (New York: Biblo & Tannen, 1933). Also Claude Lévi-Strauss, *The Savage Mind* (Chicago: Univ. of Chicago Press, 1966), especially pp. 30–3, 237–52. Sigmund Freud, *Totem and Taboo* (New York: Norton, 1952).

and Islamic Middle Ages, death continued to be regarded as the result of a deliberate personal intervention of God. No figure of "a" death appears at the deathbed, just an angel and a devil struggling over the soul escaping from the mouth of the dying. Only during the fifteenth century were the conditions ripe for a change in this image,[12] and for the appearance of what would later be called a "natural death." The dance of the dead represents this readiness. Death can now become an inevitable, intrinsic part of human life, rather than the decision of a foreign agent. Death becomes autonomous and for three centuries coexists as a separate agent with the immortal soul, with divine providence, and with angels and demons.

The Danse Macabre

In the morality plays,[13] death appears in a new costume and role. By the end of the fifteenth century, no longer just a mirror image, he assumed the leading role among the "last four things," preceding judgment, heaven, and hell.[14] Nor is he any longer just one of the four apocalyptic riders from Romanesque bas-reliefs, or the batlike Maegera who picks up souls from the cemetery of Pisa, or a mere messenger executing the orders of God. Death has become an independent figure who calls each man, woman, and child, first as a messenger from God but soon insisting on his own sovereign rights. By 1538 Hans Holbein the Younger[15] had published the first

---

[12]Robert Bossuat, *Manuel bibliographique de la littérature française du moyen âge* (Melun: Librairie d'Argences, 1951), "Danse macabre," nos. 3577–80, 7013.

[13]For the evolution of the Jederman motif see H. Lindner, *Hugo von Hoffmannstahls "Jederman" und seine Vorgänger,* dissertation, Univ. of Leipzig, 1928.

[14]Alberto Tenenti, *Il senso della morte e l'amore nella vita del Rinascimento* (Turin: Einaudi, 1957). Alberto Tenenti, *La Vie et la mort à travers l'art du XVe siècle* (Paris: Colin, 1962).

[15]Hans Holbein the Younger, *The Dance of Death: A Complete Facsimile of the Original 1538 Edition of Les Simulachres et histoires faces de la mort* (New York: Dover, 1971).

picture-book of death, which was to become a best-seller: woodcuts on the Danse Macabre.[16] The dance

---

[16]Walter Rehm, *Der Todesgedanke in der deutschen Dichtung vom Mittelalter bis zur Romantik* (Tübingen: Niemeyer, 1967), gives evidence of a major change in the image of death in literature around the year 1400 and then again around 1520. See also Edelgard Dubruck, *The Theme of Death in French Poetry of the Middle Ages and the Renaissance* (Atlantic Highlands, N.J.: Humanities Press, 1965), and L. P. Kurtz, *The Dance of Death and the Macabre Spirit in European Literature* (New York: Institute of French Studies, 1934). For the new death image of the rising middle classes of the late Middle Ages see Erna Hirsch, *Tod und Jenseits im Spätmittelalter: Zugleich ein Beitrag zur Kulturgeschichte des deutschen Búrgertums*, dissertation, Univ. of Marburg (Berlin, 1927). Specifically on the Dance of Death: Hellmut Rosenfeld, *Der mittelalterliche Totentanz: Entstehung, Entwicklung, Bedeutung* (Münster Köln: Bohlau, 1954), illustrated. Hellmut Rosenfeld, "Der Totentanz in Deutschland, Frankreich und Italien," *Littérature Moderne* 5 (1954): 62–80. Rosenfeld is the best introduction to the research and gives a detailed up-to-date bibliography. For older literature complement with H. F. Massman, *Literatur der Totentänze* (Leipzig: Weipel, 1840). See also Gert Buchheit, *Der Totentanz, seine Entstehung und Entwicklung* (Berlin: Horen, 1928), Wolfgang Stammler, *Die Totentänze des Mittelalters* (Munich: Stobbe, 1922), and James M. Clark, *The Dance of Death in the Middle Ages and the Renaissance* (Glasgow: Jackson, 1950). Stephen P. Kosaky's three volumes: *Geschichte der Totentänze*, vol. 1, *Lieferung: Anfänge der Darstellungen des Vergänglichkeitsproblems;* vol. 2, *Lieferung: Danse macabre Einleitung: Die Todesdidaktik der Vortotentanzzeit;* vol. 3, *Lieferung: Der Totentanz von heute,* Bibliotheca Humanitatis Historica, vols. 1, 5, and 7 (Budapest: Magyar Történiti Múzeum, 1936–44), contains a mine of information, quotations from ancient texts, and nearly 700 pictures (greatly reduced and badly reproduced) of the Dance of Death up to World War II. J. Saugnieux, *L'Iconographie de la mort chez les graveurs français du XVe siècle* (1974), and *Danses macabres de France et d'Espagne et leurs prolongements littéraires,* fasc. 30, Bibliothèque de la Faculté des Lettres de Lyon (Paris: Les Belles Lettres, 1972). Dietrich Briesenmeister, *Bilder des Todes* (Unterscheidheim: W. Elf, 1970): reproductions are very clear and are organized according to different themes. Consult the standard iconographies on Western Christian art: Karl Kunstle, *Ikonographie der christlicher Kunst,* 2 vols. (Freiburg: Herder, 1926–28); Émile Male, *L'Art religieux à la fin du moyen âge en France: Étude sur l'iconographie du moyen âge et sur ses sources d'inspiration* (Paris: Colin, 1908), vol. 1, chap. 2 "La Mort," p. 346 (see also the three other volumes on religious art in France). Compare Eastern iconography (Mount Athos): Dionysios of Fourna, *Manuel d'iconographie chrétienne, grècque et latine,* with introduction and notes by A. N. Didron, trans. by P. Durand from a Byzantine manuscript (1845; reprint ed., New York: B. Franklin, 1963). T. S. R. Boase, *Death in the Middle Ages: Mortality, Judgement and Remembrance* (New York: McGraw-Hill, 1972).

partners have shed their putrid flesh and turned into naked skeletons. The representation of each man as entwined with his own mortality has now changed to show his frenzied exhaustion in the grip of death painted as a force of nature. The intimate mirror-image of the "self" which had been colored by the "new devotion" of the German mystics has been replaced by a death painted as the egalitarian executioner of a law that whirls everyone along and then mows them down. From a lifelong encounter, death has turned into the event of a moment.

During the Middle Ages eternity, together with God's presence, had been immanent in history. Now death becomes the point at which linear clock-time ends and eternity meets man. The world has ceased to be a sacrament of this presence; with Luther it became the place of corruption that God saves. The proliferation of clocks symbolizes this change in consciousness. With the predominance of serial time, concern for its exact measurement, and the recognition of the simultaneity of events, a new framework for the recognition of personal identity is manufactured. The identity of the person is sought in reference to a sequence of events rather than in the completeness of one's life span. Death ceases to be the end of a whole and becomes an interruption in the sequence.[17]

Skeleton men predominate on the title pages of

---

[17]See Helmuth Plessner, "On the Relation of Time to Death," in Joseph Campbell, ed., *Papers from the Eranos Yearbooks,* vol. 3, *Man and Time,* Bollingen Series XXX (Princeton, N.J.: Princeton Univ. Press, 1957), pp. 233–63, especially p. 255. On the impact of time on the French death-image, see Richard Glasser, *Time in French Life and Thought,* trans. C. G. Pearson (Manchester: University Press, 1972), in particular p. 158 and chap. 3, "The Concept of Time in the Later Middle Ages," pp. 70–132. On the growing impact of time consciousness on the sense of finitude and death, see Alois Hahn, *Einstellungen zum Tod und ihre soziale Bedingtheit: Eine soziologische Untersuchung* (Stuttgart: Enke, 1968), especially pp. 21–84. Joost A. M. Keerloo, "The Time Sense in Psychiatry," in J. T. Fraser, ed., *The Voices of Time* (New York: Braziller, 1966), pp. 235–52, Siegfried Giedion, *Space, Time and Architecture: The Growth of a New Tradition,* 4th ed. (Cambridge, Mass.: Harvard Univ. Press, 1962).

the first fifty years of the woodcut, as naked women now predominate on magazine covers. Death holds the hourglass or strikes the tower clock.[18] Many a bell clapper was shaped like a bone. The new machine, which can make time of equal length, day and night, also puts all people under the same law. By the time of the Reformation, postmortem survival has ceased to be a transfigured continuation of life here below, and has become either a frightful punishment in the form of hell or a totally unmerited gift from God in heaven. Indwelling grace has been turned into justification by faith alone. Thus during the sixteenth century, death ceases to be conceived of primarily as a transition into the next world, and the accent is placed on the end of this life.[19] The open grave looms much larger than the doors of heaven or hell and the encounter with death has become more certain than immortality, more just than king, pope, or even God. Rather than life's aim, it has become the end of life.

The finality, imminence, and intimacy of personal death were not only part of the new sense of time but also of the emergence of a new sense of individuality. On the pilgrim's path from the Church Militant on earth to the Church Triumphant in heaven, death was experienced very much as an event that concerned both communities. Now each man faced his own and final death. Of course, once death had become such a natural force, people wanted to master it by learning the art or the skill of dying. *Ars Moriendi*, one of the first printed do-it-yourself manuals on the market, remained a best-seller in various versions for the next two hundred years. Many people learned to read by deciphering it. The most widely circulated version was published by Caxton at the Westminster press in 1491: over one hundred incunabula editions were made before 1500 from woodblocks and from movable type, under the title *Art and Craft to knowe ye well to dye*. The small folio printed in neat Goth-

---

[18]Jurgis Baltrusaitis, *Le Moyen Age fantastique: Antiquités et exotisme dans l'art gothique* (Paris: Colin, 1955).

[19]Martin Luther, interpretation of Psalm 90, WA 40/III: 485 ff.

ic letters was part of a series to instruct the "complete gentleman" in "behaviour, gentle and devout," from manipulating a table knife to conducting a conversation, from the art of weeping and blowing the nose to the art of playing chess, of praying, and of dying.

This was not a book of remote preparation for death through a virtuous life, nor a reminder to the reader of an inevitable steady decline of physical forces and the constant danger of death. It was a "how-to" book in the modern sense, a complete guide to the business of dying, a method to be learned while one was in good health and to be kept at one's fingertips for use in that inescapable hour. The book is not written for monks and ascetics but for "carnall and secular" men for whom the ministrations of the clergy were not available. It served as a model for similar instructions, often written in much less matter-of-fact spirit, by people like Savonarola, Luther, and Jeremy Taylor. Men felt responsible for the expression their face would show in death.[20] Kunstler has shown that about this very time an unprecedented approach was developed in the painting of human faces: the Western portrait of countenance, which tries to represent much more than just the likeness of facial traits. The first portraits, in fact, represent princes and were executed immediately after their death, from memory, in order to render the individu-

---

[20]The response to "natural" death was a profound transformation of behavior at the hour of death. For contemporary literature, see Mary Catherine O'Connor, *The Art of Dying Well: The Development of the Ars Moriendi* (New York: AMS Press, 1966). L. Klein, *Die Bereitung zum Sterben: Studien zu den evangelischen Sterbebüchern des 16. Jahrhunderts,* dissertation, Univ. of Göttingen, 1958. For customs see Placidus Berger, "Religiöser Brauchtum im Umkreis der Sterbeliturgie in Deutschland," *Zeitschrift fur Missionswissenschaft und Religionswissenschaft* 5 (1948): 108–248. See also Manfred Bambeck, "Tod und Unsterblichkeit: Studien zum Lebensgefühl der französischen Renaissance nach dem Werke Ronsarde," ms. dissertation, Univ. of Frankfurt, 1954. Hildegard Reifschneider, "Die Vorstellung des Todes und des Jenseits in der geistlichen Literatur des XII Jh.," ms. dissertation, Univ. of Tübingen, 1948. Eberhard Klass, *Die Schilderung des Sterbens im mittelhochedeutschen Epos: Ein Beitrag zur mittelhochdeutschen Stilgeschichte,* dissertation, Univ. of Greifswald, 1931.

al, atemporal personality of the deceased ruler present at his state funeral. Early Renaissance humanists wanted to remember their dead, not as ghouls or ghosts, saints or symbols, but as a continuing, personal, historical presence.[21]

In popular devotion a new kind of curiosity about the afterlife developed. Fantastic horror stories about dead bodies and artistic representations of purgatory both multiplied.[22] The grotesque concern of the seventeenth century with ghosts and souls underscores the growing anxiety of a culture faced with the call of death rather than the judgment of God.[23] In many parts of the Christian world the dance of death became a standard decoration in the entrance of parish churches. The Spaniards brought the skeleton man to America, where he fused with the Aztec idol of death. Their mestizo offspring,[24] on its rebound to Europe, influenced the face of death throughout the Hapsburg Empire from Holland to the Tyrol. After the Reformation, European death became and remained macabre.

Simultaneously, medical folk-practices multiplied, all designed to help people meet their death with dignity as individuals. New superstitious devices were developed so that one might recognize whether

---

[21]Gustav Kunstler, "Das Bildnis Rudolf des Stifters, Herzogs von Österreich, und seine Funktion," excerpt from *Mitteilungen der Österreichischen Galerie 1972* (Vienna: Kunsthistoriches Museum, 1972), about the very first such portrait.

[22]G. and M. Vovelle, "La Mort et l'au-delà en Provence d'après les autels des âmes du purgatoire: XVe-XXe siècles," *Cahiers des Annales* 29 (1970): 1602–34. Howard R. Patch, *The Other World According to Descriptions in Medieval Literature* (Cambridge, Mass.: Harvard Univ. Press, 1950).

[23]For the "judgment" in the history of religions, see Sources Orientales, *Le Jugement des morts* (Paris: Seuil, 1962); Leopold Kretzenbacher, *Die Seelenwaage: Zur religiösen Idee vom Jenseitsgericht auf der Schicksalwaage in Hochreligion, Bildkunst und Volksglaube* (Klagenfurt: Landesmuseums für Kärten, 1958).

[24]Merlin H. Forster, ed., *La muerte en la poesía mexicana: Prólogo y selección de Merlin Forster* (Mexico: Editorial Diogenes, 1970). Emir Rodríguez Monegal, "Death as a Key to Mexican Reality in the Works of Octavio Paz," mimeographed, Yale Univ., n.d. (about 1973).

one's sickness required the acceptance of approaching death or some kind of treatment. If the flower thrown into the fountain of the sanctuary drowned, it was useless to spend money on remedies. People tried to be ready when death came, to have the steps well learned for the last dance. Remedies against a painful agony multiplied, but most of them were still to be performed under the conscious direction of the dying, who played a new role and played it consciously. Children could help a mother or father to die, but only if they did not hold them back by crying. A person was supposed to indicate when he wanted to be lowered from his bed onto the earth which would soon engulf him, and when the prayers were to start. But bystanders knew that they were to keep the doors open to make it easy for death to come, to avoid noise so as not to frighten death away, and finally to turn their eyes respectfully away from the dying man in order to leave him alone during this most personal event.[25]

Neither priest nor doctor was expected to assist the poor man in typical fifteenth- and sixteenth-century death.[26] In principle, medical writers recognized two opposite services the physician could perform. He could either assist healing or help the coming of an easy and speedy death. It was his duty to recognize the *facies hippocratica*,[27] the special traits which in-

---

[25]In rural areas these customs live on: Arnold van Gennep, *Manuel de folklore français contemporain*, vol. 1, *Du berceau à la tombe* (Paris: Picard, 1943–46). Lenz Kriss-Rettenbeck, "Tod und Heilserwartung," in *Bilder und Zeichen religiösen Volksglaubens* (Munich: Callwey, 1963), pp. 49–56. See articles by Paul Geiger, on "Sterbegaläute," "Sterben," "Sterbender," "Sterbekerze," "Tod," "Tod ansagen," "Tote (der)," "Totenbahre," in *Handwörterbuch des deutschen Aberglaubens* (Berlin: W. de Gruyter, 1936–37), vol. 8. Albert Freybe, *Das alte deutsche Leichenmahl in seiner Art und Entartung* (Gütersloh: Bertelsmann, 1909), pp. 5–86.

[26]For an introduction to the function of the Catholic priest at the deathbed, see C. Ruch, "Extrême onction," in *Dictionnaire de Théologie Catholique* (1939), 5, pt. 2:1927–85. Henri Rondet, "Extrême onction," in *Dictionnaire de Spiritualité* (1960), 4:2189–2200.

[27]Magnus Schmid, "Zum Phänomen der Leiblichkeit in der Antike dargestellt an der 'Facies Hippocratica,'" *Sudhoffs Archiv*, suppl. 7, 1966, pp. 168–77. Karl Sudhoff, "Eine kleine deutsche

dicated that the patient was already in the grip of death. In healing as in withdrawal, the doctor was anxious to work hand-in-glove with nature. The question whether medicine ever could "prolong" life was heatedly disputed in the medical schools of Palermo, Fez, and even Paris. Many Arab and Jewish doctors denied this power outright, and declared such an attempt to interfere with the order of nature to be blasphemous.[28]

Vocational zeal tempered by philosophical resignation comes through clearly in the writings of Paracelsus.[29] "Nature knows the boundaries of her course. According to her own appointed term, she confers upon each of her creatures its proper life span, so that its energies are consumed during the time that elapses between the moment of its birth and its predestined end. . . . A man's death is nothing but the end of his daily work, an expiration of air, the consummation of his innate balsamic self-curing power, the extinction of the rational light of nature, and a great separation of the three: body, soul, and spirit. Death is a return to the womb." Without excluding transcendence, death has become a natural phenomenon, no longer requiring that blame be placed on some evil agent.

The new image of death helped to reduce the human body to an object. Up to this time, the corpse had been considered something quite unlike other things: it was treated almost like a person. The law recognized its standing: the dead could sue and be sued by the living, and criminal proceedings against the dead were common. Pope Urban VIII, who had been poisoned by his successor, was dug up, solemnly judged a simonist, had his right hand cut off, and was

---

Todesprognosik," *Archiv für Geschichte der Medizin* 5 (1911): 240, and "Abermal eine deutsche Lebens- und Todesprognostic," *ibid.*, 6 (1911): 231.

[28]Joshua O. Leibowitz, "A Responsum of Maimonides Concerning the Termination of Life," *Koroth* (Jerusalem) 5 (September 1963): 1–2.

[29]Paracelsus, *Selected Writings,* trans, Norbert Guterman, Bollingen Series XXVIII (Princeton, N.J.: Princeton Univ. Press, 1969).

thrown into the Tiber. After being hanged as a thief, a man might still have his head cut off for being a traitor. The dead could also be called to witness. The widow could still repudiate her husband by putting the keys and his purse on his casket. Even today the executor acts in the name of the dead, and we still speak of the "desecration" of a grave or the secularization of a public cemetery when it is turned into a park. The appearance of natural death was necessary for the corpse to be deprived of much of its legal standing.[30]

The arrival of natural death also prepared the way for new attitudes towards death and disease which became common in the late seventeenth century. During the Middle Ages, the human body had been sacred; now the physician's scalpel had access to the corpse itself.[31] Its dissection had been considered by the humanist Gerson to be "a sacrilegious profanation, a useless cruelty exercised by the living against the dead."[32] But at the same time that Everyman's Death began to emerge in person in the morality plays, the corpse first appeared as a teaching

---

[30]Heinrich Brunner, *Deutsche Rechtsgeschichte* (Berlin: Von Duncker & Humbolt, 1961), 1:254 ff. Paul Fischer, *Strafen und sichernde Massnahmen gegen Tote im germanischen und deutschen Recht* (Düsseldorf: Nolte, 1936). H. Fehr, "Tod und Teufel im alten Recht," *Zeitschrift der Savigny Stiftung fur Rechtsgeschichte* 67 (1950): 50–75. Paul Geiger, "Leiche," in *Handwörterbuch des deutschen Aberglaubens* (Berlin: W. de Gruyter, 1932–33), vol 5. Karl König, "Die Behandlung der Toten in Frankreich im späteren Mittelalter und zu Beginn der Neuzeit (1350–1550)," ms. dissertation, Univ. of Leipzig, 1921. Hans von Hentig, *Der nekrotrope Mensch: Vom Totenglauben zur morbiden Totennähe* (Stuttgart: Enke, 1964). Paul-J. Doll, "Les Droits de la science après la mort," *Diogène*, no. 75, July–September 1971, pp. 124–42.

[31]The contrast appears clearly when Loren C. MacKinney, *Medical Illustrations in Medieval Manuscripts* (Berkeley: Univ. of California Press, 1965), is compared with Millard Meiss, *Painting in Florence and Siena after the Black Death: The Arts, Religion and Society in the Mid-Fourteenth Century* (Princeton, N.J.: Princeton Univ. Press, 1951). Art, liberated from the need to represent dogma, now shows the human figure, its actions, and even the dead things which surround it as intimately interwoven in the representation of the fleeting moment (*Vergänglichkeit*).

[32]Maurice Bariety and Charles Coury, "La Dissection," in *Historie de la médecine* (Paris: Fayard, 1963), pp. 409–11.

object in the amphitheater of the Renaissance university. When the first authorized public dissection took place in Montpellier in 1375, this new learned activity was declared obscene, and the performance could not be repeated for several years. A generation later, permission was given for one corpse a year to be dissected within the borders of the German Empire. At the University of Bologna, also, one body was dissected each year just before Christmas, and the ceremony was inaugurated by a procession, accompanied by exorcisms, and took three days. During the fifteenth century, the University of Lérida in Spain was entitled to the corpse of one criminal every three years, to be dissected in the presence of a notary assigned by the Inquisition. In England in 1540, the faculties of the universities were authorized to claim four corpses a year from the hangman. Attitudes changed so rapidly that by 1561 the Venetian Senate ordered the hangman to take instruction from Dr. Fallopius in order to provide him with corpses well suited for "anatomizing." Rembrandt painted "Dr. Tulp's Lesson" in 1632. Public dissection became a favored subject for paintings and, in the Netherlands, a common event at carnivals. The first step towards surgery on television and in the movies had been taken. The physician had advanced his knowledge of anatomy and his power to exhibit his skill, but both were disproportionate to an advance in his ability to heal. Medical rituals helped to orient, repress, or allay the fear and anguish generated by a death that had become macabre. The anatomy of Vesalius rivaled Holbein's Danse Macabre somewhat as scientific sex-guides now rival *Playboy* and *Penthouse* magazines.

Bourgeois Death

Baroque death counterpointed an aristocratically organized heaven.[33] The church vault might depict a

---

[33]Hermann Bauer, *Der Himmel in Rokoko: Das Fresko im deutschen Kirchenraum in 18. Jahrhundert* (Munich: Pustet, 1965).

last judgment with separate spaces reserved for savages, commoners, and nobles, but the Dance of Death beneath depicted the mower who used his scythe regardless of post or rank. Precisely because macabre equality belittled worldly privilege, it also made it more legitimate.[34] However, with the rise of the bourgeois family,[35] equality in death came to an end: those who could afford it began to pay to keep death away.

Francis Bacon was the first to speak about the prolongation of life as a new task for physicians. He divided medicine into three offices: "First, the preservation of health, second, the cure of disease, and third, the prolongation of life," and extolled the "third part of medicine, regarding the prolongation of life: this is a new part, and deficient, although the most noble of all." The medical profession did not even consider facing this task, until, some one hundred and fifty years later, there appeared a host of clients who were anxious to pay for the attempt. This was a new type of rich man who refused to die in retirement and insisted on being carried away by death from natural exhaustion while still on the job. He refused to accept death unless he was in good health in an active old age. Montaigne had already ridiculed such people as exceptionally conceited:

---

[34]Reflection of death in 17th and 18th century literature: Richard Sexau, *Der Tod in deutschen Drama des 17. und 18. Jahrhunderts: Von Griphius bis zum Sturm und Drang* (Bern: Francke, 1906). Friedrich-Wilhelm Eggebert, *Das Problem des Todes in der deutschen Lyrik des 17. Jahrhunderts* (Leipzig, 1931). W. M. Thompson, *Der Tod in der englische Lyrik des 17. Jahrhunderts* (Breslau: Priebatsch, 1935).

[35]Ariès, "La mort inversée": "In the late Middle Ages (in opposition to the first Middle Ages, the age of Roland, which lives on in the peasants of Tolstoy) and the Renaissance, a man insisted upon participating in his own death because he saw in it an exceptional moment—a moment which gave his individuality its definitive form. He was only the master of his life to the extent that he was the master of his death. His death belonged to him, and to him alone. From the 17th century onward, one began to abdicate sole sovereignty over life, as well as over death. These matters came to be shared with the family which had previously been excluded from the serious decisions; all decisions had been made by the dying person, alone and with full knowledge of his impending death."

"'Tis the last and extreme form of dying . . . what an idle conceit is it to expect to die of a decay of strength which is the effect of the extremest age, and to propose to ourselves no shorter lease on life . . . as if it were contrary to nature to see a man break his neck with a fall, be drowned by shipwreck, be snatched away with pleurisy or the plague . . . we ought to call natural death that which is general, common and universal."[36] Such people were few in his time; soon their numbers would increase. The preacher expecting to go to heaven, the philosopher denying the existence of the soul, and the merchant wanting to see his capital double once more were all in agreement that the only death that accorded with nature was one which would overtake them at their desks.[37]

There is no evidence to show that the age-specific life expectancy of most people in their sixties had increased by the middle of the eighteenth century, but there is no doubt that new technology had made it possible for the old and rich to hang on while doing what they had done in middle age. The pampered could stay on the job because their living and working conditions had eased. The Industrial Revolution had begun to create employment opportunities for the weak, sickly, and old. Sedentary work, hitherto rare, had come into its own.[38] Rising entrepreneurship and capitalism favored the boss who had had the time to accumulate capital and experience. Roads had improved: a general affected by gout could now command a battle from his wagon, and decrepit dip-

---

[36]Michel de Montaigne, *Essays*, bk. 1, chap. 57.

[37]G. Peignot, *Choix de testaments anciens et modernes, remarquables par leur importance, leur singularité ou leur bizarrerie*, 2 vols. (Paris: Renouard, 1829). Michel Vovelle, *Mourir autrefois: Attitudes collectives devant la mort aux XVIIe et XVIIIe siècles* (Paris: Archives Gallimard-Julliard, 1974), and *Piété baroque et déchristianisation en Provence au XVIIIe siècle: Les Attitudes devant la mort d'après les clauses des testaments* (Paris: Plon, 1974). Frederick Pollock and Frederic W. Maitland, "The Last Will," in *The History of the English Law Before the Time of Edward I* (Cambridge: University Press, 1968), vol. 1, chap. 6, pp. 314–56.

[38]Ariés, "Les Techniques de la mort."

lomats could travel from London to Vienna or Moscow. Centralized nation-states increased the need for scribes and an enlarged bourgeoisie. The new and small class of old men had a greater chance of survival because their lives at home, on the street, and at work had become physically less demanding. Aging had become a way of capitalizing life. Years at the desk, either at the counter or the school bench, began to bear interest on the market. The young of the middle class, whether gifted or not, were now for the first time sent to school, thus allowing the old to stay on the job. The bourgeoisie who could afford to eliminate "social death" by avoiding retirement, created "childhood" to keep their young under control.[39]

Along with the economic status of the old, the value of their bodily functions increased. In the sixteenth century "a young wife is death to an old man," and in the seventeenth, "old men who play with young maids dance with death." At the court of Louis XIV the old lecher was a laughingstock; by the time of the Congress of Vienna he had turned into an object of envy. To die while courting one's grandson's mistress became the symbol of a desirable end.

A new myth about the social value of the old was developed. Primitive hunters, gatherers, and nomads had usually killed them, and peasants had put them into the back room,[40] but now the patriarch appeared as a literary ideal. Wisdom was attributed to him just because of his age. It first became tolerable and then appropriate that the elderly should attend with solici-

---

[39]Philippe Ariés, *Centuries of Childhood: A Social History of Family Life* (New York: Knopf, 1962), chap. 2.

[40]Killing the aged was a widespread custom until recent times. John Koty, *Die Behandlung der Alten und Kranken bei den Naturvölkern* (Stuttgart: Hirschfeld, 1934). Will-Eich Peuckert, "Altentötung," in *Handwörterbuch der Sage: Namens des Verbandes der Vereine für Volkskunde* (Gottingen: Vandenhoeck & Ruprecht, 1961). J. Wisse, *Selbstmord und Todesfurcht bei den Naturvölkern* (Zutphen: Thieme, 1933). Infanticide remained important enough to influence population trends until the 9th century. Emily R. Coleman, "L'Infanticide dans le haut moyen âge," trans. A. Chamoux, *Annales Économies, Sociétés, Civilisations,* 1974, no. 2, pp. 315–35.

tude to the rituals deemed necessary to keep up their tottering bodies. No physician was yet in attendance to take on this task, which lay beyond the competence claimed by apothecary or herbalist, barber or surgeon, university-trained doctor or traveling quack. But it was this peculiar demand that helped to create a new kind of self-styled healer.[41]

Formerly, only king or pope had been under an obligation to remain in command until the day of his death. They alone consulted the faculties: the Arabs from Salerno in the Middle Ages, or the Renaissance men from Padua or Montpellier. Kings, however, kept court physicians to do what barbers did for the commoner: bleed them and purge them, and in addition, protect them from poisons. Kings neither set out to live longer than others, nor expected their personal physicians to give special dignity to their declining years. In contrast, the new class of old men saw in death the absolute price for absolute economic value.[42] The aging accountant wanted a doctor who

---

[41]Erwin H. Ackerknecht, "Death in the History of Medicine," *Bulletin of the History of Medicine* 42 (1968): 19–23. Death remained a marginal problem in medical literature from the old Greeks until Giovanni Maria Lancisi (1654–1720) during the first decade of the eighteenth century. Then quite suddenly the "signs of death" acquired extraordinary importance. Apparent death became a major evil feared by the Enlightenment. Margot Augener, "Scheintod als medizinisches Problem im 18. Jahrhundert," *Mitteilungen zur Geschichte der Medizin,* nos. 6 and 7, 1967. The same philosophers who were the minority which positively denied the survival of a soul also developed a secularized fear of hell which might threaten them if they were buried while only apparently dead. Philanthropists fighting for those in danger of apparent death founded societies dedicated to the succor of the drowning or burning, and tests were developed for making sure that they had died. Elizabeth Thomson, "The Role of the Physician in Human Societies of the 18th Century," *Bulletin of the History of Medicine* 37 (1963): 43–51. One of these tests consisted of blowing with a trumpet into the dead man's ear. The hysteria about apparent death disappeared with the French Revolution as suddenly as it had appeared at the dawn of the century. Doctors began to be concerned with reanimation a century before they were employed in the hope of prolonging the life of the old.

[42]Theodor W. Adorno, *Minima Moralia: Reflexionen aus dem beschädigten Leben* (Frankfurt am Main: Suhrkamp, 1970).

would drive away death; when the end approached, he wanted to be formally "given up" by his doctor and to be served his last repast with the special bottle reserved for the occasion. The role of the "valetudinarian" was thereby created, and with genteel decrepitude, the eighteenth-century groundwork was laid for the economic power of the contemporary physician.

The ability to survive longer, the refusal to retire before death, and the demand for medical assistance in an incurable condition had joined forces to give rise to a new concept of sickness: the type of health to which old age could aspire. In the years just before the French Revolution this had become the health of the rich and the powerful; within a generation chronic disease became fashionable for the young and pretentious, consumptive features[43] the sign of premature wisdom, and the need for travel into warm climates a claim to genius. Medical care for protracted ailments, even though they might lead to untimely death, had become a mark of distinction.

By contrast, a reverse judgment now could be made on the ailments of the poor, and the ills from which they had always died could be defined as untreated sickness. It did not matter at all if the treatment doctors could provide for these ills had any effect on the progress of the sickness; the lack of such treatment began to mean that they were condemned to die an unnatural death, an idea that fitted the bourgeois image of the poor as uneducated and unproductive. From now on the ability to die a "natural" death was reserved to one social class: those who could afford to die as patients.

Health became the privilege of waiting for timely death, no matter what medical service was needed for this purpose. In an earlier epoch, death had carried the hourglass. In woodcuts, both skeleton and onlooker grin when the victim refuses death. Now the

---

[43]E. Ebstein, "Die Lungenschwindsucht in der Weltliteratur," *Zeitschrift für Bücherfreunde* 5 (1913).

middle class seized the clock and employed doctors to tell death when to strike.[44] The Enlightenment attributed a new power to the doctor, without being able to verify whether or not he had acquired any new influence over the outcome of dangerous sickness.

Clinical Death

The French Revolution marked a short interruption in the medicalization of death. Its ideologues believed that untimely death would not strike in a society built on its triple ideal. But the doctor's newly acquired *clinical* eyeglasses made him look at death in a new perspective. Whereas the merchants of the eighteenth century had determined the outlook on death with the help of the charlatans they employed and paid, now the clinicians began to shape the public's vision. We have seen death turn from God's call into a "natural" event and later into a "force of nature"; in a further mutation it had turned into an "untimely" event when it came to those who were not both healthy and old. Now it had become the outcome of specific diseases certified by the doctor.[45]

Death had paled into a metaphorical figure, and killer diseases had taken his place. The general force of nature that had been celebrated as "death" had turned into a host of specific causations of clinical demise. Many "deaths" now roamed the world. A number of book plates from private libraries of late nineteenth-century physicians show the doctor battling with personified diseases at the bedside of his patient. The hope of doctors to control the outcome of specific diseases gave rise to the myth that they had

---

[44]Alfred Scott Warthin, "The Physician of the Dance of Death," *Annals of Medical History* (new series) 2 (July 1930): 350–71; 2 (September 1930): 453–69; 2 (November 1930): 697–710; 3 (January 1931): 75–109; 3 (March 1931): 134–65. Deals exclusively with the physician in the Dance of Death. Werner Block, *Der Arzt und der Tod in Bildern aus sechs Jahrhunderten* (Stuttgart: Enke, 1966), studies the doctor's encounter with death in and outside a formal dance.

[45]See above, note 130, p. 71.

power over death. The new powers attributed to the profession gave rise to the new status of the clinician.[46]

While the city physician became a clinician, the country physician became first sedentary and then a member of the local elite. At the time of the French Revolution he had still belonged to the traveling folk. The surplus of army surgeons from the Napoleonic wars came home with a vast experience, looking for a living. Military men trained on the battlefield, they soon became the first resident healers in France, Italy, and Germany. The simple people did not quite trust their techniques and staid burghers were shocked by their rough ways, but still they found clients because of their reputation among veterans of the Napoleonic wars. They sent their sons to the new medical schools springing up in the cities, and these upon their return created the role of the country doctor, which remained unchanged up to the time of World War II. They derived a steady income from playing the family doctor to the middle class who could well afford them. A few of the city or town rich acquired prestige by living as patients of famous clinicians, but in the early nineteenth century a much more serious competition for the town doctor still came from the medical technicians of old—the midwife, the tooth-puller, the veterinarian, the barber, and sometimes the public nurse. Notwithstanding the newness of his role and resistance to it from above and below, the European country doctor, by mid-century, had become a member of the middle class. He earned enough from playing lackey to a squire, was family friend to other notables, paid occasional visits to the lowly sick, and sent his complicated cases to his clinical colleague in town. While "timely" death had originated in the emerging class consciousness of the bourgeois, "clinical" death originated in the emerging professional consciousness of the new, scientifically trained doctor.

---

[46]Richard H. Shryock, *The Development of Modern Medicine: An Interpretation of the Social and Scientific Factors Involved*, 2nd ed. (New York: Knopf, 1947).

Henceforth, a timely death with clinical symptoms became the ideal of middle-class doctors,[47] and it was soon to become incorporated into the aspirations of trade unions.

Trade Union Claims to a Natural Death

In our century a valetudinarian's death while undergoing treatment by clinically trained doctors came to be perceived, for the first time, as a civil right. Old-age medical care was written into union contracts. The capitalist privilege of natural extinction from exhaustion in a director's chair gave way to the proletarian demand for health services during retirement. The bourgeois hope of continuing as a dirty old man in the office was ousted by the dream of an active sex life on social security in a retirement village. Lifelong care for every clinical condition soon became a peremptory demand for access to a natural death. Lifelong institutional medical care had become a service that society owed all its members.

"Natural death" now appeared in dictionaries. One major German encyclopedia published in 1909 defines it by means of contrast: "Abnormal death is opposed to natural death because it results from sickness, violence, or mechanical and chronic disturbances." A reputable dictionary of philosophical concepts states that "natural death comes without previous sickness, without definable specific cause." It was this macabre hallucinatory death-concept that became intertwined with the concept of social progress. Legally valid claims to equality in clinical death spread the contradictions of bourgeois individualism among the working class. The right to a natural death was formulated as a claim to equal consumption of medical services, rather than as a freedom from the evils of industrial work or as a new liberty and power for self-care. This unionized concept of an "equal

---

[47] Hildegard Steingiesser, *Was die Ärzte aller Zeiten vom Sterben wussten,* Arbeiten der deutsch-nordischen Gesellschaft für Geschichte der Medizin, der Zahnheilkunde und der Naturwissenschaften (Greifswald: Univ. Verlag Ratsbuchhandlung L. Bamberg, 1936).

clinical death" is thus the inverse of the ideal proposed in the National Assembly of Paris in 1792: it is a deeply medicalized ideal.

First of all, this new image of death endorses new levels of social control. Society has become responsible for preventing each man's death: treatment, effective or not, can be made into a duty. Any fatality occurring without medical treatment is liable to become a coroner's case. The encounter with a doctor becomes almost as inexorable as the encounter with death. I know of a woman who tried, unsuccessfully, to kill herself. She was brought to the hospital in a coma, with a bullet lodged in her spine. Using heroic measures the surgeon kept her alive, and he considers her case a success: she lives, but she is totally paralyzed; he no longer has to worry about her ever attempting suicide again.

Our new image of death also befits the industrial ethos.[48] The good death has irrevocably become that of the standard consumer of medical care. Just as at the turn of the century all men were defined as pupils, born into original stupidity and standing in need of eight years of schooling before they could enter productive life, today they are stamped from birth as patients who need all kinds of treatment if they want to lead life the right way. Just as compulsory educational consumption came to be used as a device to obviate concern about work, so medical consumption became a device to alleviate unhealthy work, dirty cities, and nerve-racking transportation.[49] What need is there to worry about a murderous environment when doctors are industrially equipped to act as life-savers!

Finally, "death under compulsory care" encourages the re-emergence of the most primitive delusions

---

[48]Bernard Ronze, "L'Antitragique ou l'homme qui perd sa mort," *Études*, November 1974, pp. 511–28, argues that the endeavor to program death is an attempt to sap the human capacity for hope and anguish, for solitude and transcendence.

[49]Siegfried Giedion, *Mechanization Takes Command: A Contribution to Anonymous History* (New York: Norton, 1969). On mechanization and death, see pp. 209–40.

about the causes of death. As we have seen, primitive people do not die of their own death, they do not carry finitude in their bones, and they are still close to the subjective immortality of the beast. Among them, death always requires a supernatural explanation, somebody to blame: the curse of an enemy, the spell of a magician, the breaking of the yarn in the hands of the Parcae, or God dispatching his angel of death. In the dance with his or her mirror-image, European death emerged as an agent independent of another's will, an inexorable force of nature that men and women had to face on their own. The imminence of death was an exquisite and constant reminder of the fragility and tenderness of life. During the late Middle Ages, the discovery of "natural" death became one of the mainsprings of European lyric and drama. But the same imminence of death, once perceived as an extrinsic threat coming from nature, became a major challenge for the emerging engineer. If the civil engineer had learned to manage earth, and the pedagogue-become-educator to manage knowledge, why should the biologist-physician not manage death?[50] When the doctor contrived to step between humanity and death, the latter lost the immediacy and intimacy gained four hundred years earlier. Death that had lost face and shape had lost *its* dignity.

The change in the doctor-death relationship can be well illustrated by following the iconographic treatment of this theme.[51] In the age of the Dance of Death, the physician is rare. In the only picture I have located in which death treats the doctor as a colleague, he has taken an old man by one hand, while in the other he carries a glass of urine, and seems to be asking the physician to confirm his diagnosis. In the age of the Dance of Death, the skeleton man makes the doctor the main butt of his jokes. In

---

[50]Alfred Adler, "Ein Beitrag zur Psychologie der Berufswahl," in Alfred Weber and Carl Furtmüller, eds. *Heilen und Bilden* (Frankfurt: Fischer, 1973).

[51]See especially Block, *Der Arzt und der Tod;* Warthin, "The Physician of the Dance of Death"; Briesenmeister, *Bilder des Todes.*

the earlier period, while death still wore some flesh, he asks the doctor to confirm in the latter's own mirror-image what he thought he knew about man's innards. Later, as a fleshless skeleton, he teases the doctor about his impotence, jokes about or rejects his honoraria, offers medicine as pernicious as that the physician dispensed, and treats the doctor as just one more common mortal by snatching him into the dance. Baroque death seems to intrude constantly into the doctor's activities, making fun of him while he sells his wares at a fair, interrupting his consultation, transforming his medicine bottles into hourglasses, or taking the doctor's place on a visit to the pesthouse. In the eighteenth century a new motif appears: death seems to enjoy teasing the physician about his pessimistic diagnoses, abandoning those sick persons whom the doctor has condemned, and dragging the doctor off to the tomb while leaving the patient alive. Until the nineteenth century, death deals always with the doctor or with the sick, usually taking the initiative in the action. The contestants are at opposite ends of the sickbed. Only after clinical sickness and clinical death had developed considerably do we find the first pictures in which the doctor assumes the initiative and interposes himself between his patient and death. We have to wait until after World War I before we see physicians wrangling with the skeleton, tearing a young woman from its embrace, and wresting the scythe from death's hand. By 1930 a smiling white-coated man is rushing against a whimpering skeleton and crushing it like a fly with two volumes of Marle's *Lexicon of Therapy*. In other pictures, the doctor raises one hand and wards off death while holding up the arms of a young woman whom death grips by the feet. Max Klinger represents the physician clipping the feathers of a winged giant. Others show the physician locking the skeleton into prison or even kicking its bony bottom. Now the doctor rather than the patient struggles with death. As in primitive cultures, somebody can again be blamed when death triumphs. This somebody is no longer a person with the face of a witch, an ancestor, or a god, but the enemy in the shape of a social force.[52] Today, when defense against death is included in social security, the culprit lurks within society. The culprit might be the class enemy who deprives the worker of sufficient medical care, the doctor who refuses to make a night visit, the multinational concern that raises the price of medicine, the capitalist or revisionist government that has lost control over its medicine men, or the administrator who partly trains physicians at the University of Delhi and then drains them off to London. The witch-hunt that was traditional at the death of a tribal chief is being modernized. For every premature or clinically unnecessary death, somebody or some body can be found who irresponsibly delayed or prevented a medical intervention.

Much of the progress of social legislation during the first half of the twentieth century would have been impossible without the revolutionary use of such an industrially graven death-image. Neither the support necessary to agitate for such legislation nor guilt feelings strong enough to enforce its enactment could have been aroused. But the claim to equal medical nurturing towards an equal kind of death has also served to consolidate the dependence of our contemporaries on a limitlessly expanding industrial system.

Death Under Intensive Care

We cannot fully understand the deeply rooted structure of our social organization unless we see in it a multifaceted exorcism of all forms of evil death. Our major institutions constitute a gigantic defense program waging war on behalf of "humanity" against death-dealing agencies and classes.[53] This is a total

---

[52]I have selected these examples from among hundreds of reproductions collected by Valentina Borremans in Cuernavaca, all representing the traits and gestures of anthropomorphic death.

[53]For a bibliography on death in contemporary society consult above, notes 186 (p. 91), 188 (p. 92), 191 (p. 92), 207 (p. 97), 209 (p. 97). Also John McKnight, "A Bibliography of 225 Items of Suggested Readings for a Course on Death in Modern Society in a

war. Not only medicine but also welfare, international relief, and development programs are enlisted in this struggle. Ideological bureaucracies of all colors join the crusade. Revolution, repression, and even civil and international wars are justified in order to defeat the dictators or capitalists who can be blamed for the wanton creation and tolerance of sickness and death.[54]

Curiously, death became the enemy to be defeated at precisely the moment at which megadeath came upon the scene. Not only the image of "unnecessary" death is new, but also our image of the end of the world.[55] Death, the end of *my* world, and apocalypse, the end of *the* world, are intimately related; our attitude towards both has clearly been deeply affected by the atomic situation. The apocalypse has ceased to be just a mythological conjecture

---

Theological Perspective," mimeographed, 1973, lists contemporary Christian writings on death in an industrial society. John Riley, Jr., and Robert W. Habenstein, "Death: 1. Death and Bereavement; 2. The Social Organization of Death," in *International Encyclopedia of the Social Sciences* (New York: Macmillan, 1968), 4: 19–28. Joel J. Vernick, *Selected Bibliography on Death and Dying,* U.S. Department of Health, Education and Welfare, Public Health Service, National Institutes of Health, 1971. Complements Kalish and Kutscher.

[54]Werner Fuchs, *Todesbilder in der modernen Gesellschaft,* denies that death is repressed in modern society. Geoffrey Gorer, *Death, Grief and Mourning* (New York: Doubleday, 1965): Gorer's thesis that death has taken the place of sex as the principal taboo seems to Fuchs unfounded and misleading. The thesis of death repression is usually promoted by people of profoundly anti-industrial persuasions for the purpose of demonstrating the ultimate powerlessness of the industrial enterprise in the face of death. Talk about death repression is used with insistence to construct apologies in favor of God and the afterlife. The fact that people have to die is taken as proof that they will never autonomously control reality. Fuchs interprets all theories that deny the quality of death as relics of a primitive past. He considers as scientific only those corresponding to his idea of a modern social structure. His image of contemporary death is a result of his study of the language used in German obituaries. He believes that what is called the "repression" of death is due to a lack of effective acceptance of the increasingly general belief in death as an unquestionable and final end.

[55]The irrational approach of a society in dealing with death is reflected in its inability to deal with apocalypse. Klaus Koch, *Ratlos vor der Apokalyptik* (Gütersloh: Mohn, 1970).

and has become a real contingency. Instead of being due to the will of God, or man's guilt, or the laws of nature, Armageddon has become a possible consequence of man's direct decision. Cobalt, like hydrogen bombs, creates an illusion of control over death. Medicalized social rituals represent one aspect of social control by means of the self-frustrating war against death.

Malinowski[56] has argued that death among primitive people threatens the cohesion and therefore the survival of the whole group. It triggers an explosion of fear and irrational expressions of defense. Group solidarity is saved by making out of the natural event a social ritual. The death of a member thereby becomes an occasion for an exceptional celebration. The dominance of industry has disrupted and often dissolved most traditional bonds of solidarity. The impersonal rituals of industrialized medicine create an ersatz unity of mankind. They tie all its members into a pattern of "desirable" death by proposing hospital death as the goal of economic development. The myth of progress of all people towards the same kind of death diminishes the feeling of guilt on the part of the "haves" by transforming the ugly deaths that the "have-nots" die into the result of present underdevelopment, which ought to be remedied by further expansion of medical institutions.

Of course, medicalized[57] death has a different function in highly industrialized societies than it has in mainly rural nations. Within an industrial society, medical intervention in everyday life does not change the prevailing image of health and death, but rather caters to it. It diffuses the death-image of the medicalized elite among the masses and reproduces it for

---

[56]Bronislav Malinowski, "Death and the Reintegration of the Group," in *Magic, Science and Religion* (New York: Doubleday, 1949), pp. 47–53.

[57]Eric J. Cassel, "Dying in a Technical Society," *Hastings Center Studies* 2 (May 1974): 31–36: "There has been a shift of death from within the moral order to the technical order. . . . I do not believe that men were inherently more moral in the past when the moral order predominated over the technical."

future generations. But when "death prevention" is applied outside of a cultural context in which consumers religiously prepare themselves for hospital deaths, the growth of hospital-based medicine inevitably constitutes a form of imperialist intervention. A sociopolitical image of death is imposed; people are deprived of their traditional vision of what constitutes health and death. The self-image that gives cohesion to their culture is dissolved, and atomized individuals can now be incorporated into an international mass of highly "socialized" health consumers. The expectation of medicalized death hooks the rich on unlimited insurance payments and lures the poor into a gilded deathtrap. The contradictions of bourgeois individualism are corroborated by the inability of people to die with any possibility of a realistic attitude towards death.[58] The customs man guarding the frontier between Upper Volta and Mali explained to me this importance of death in relation to health. I wanted to know from him how people along the Niger could understand each other, though almost every village spoke a different tongue. For him this had nothing to do with language: "As long as people cut the prepuce of their boys the way we do, and die our death, we can understand them well."

In many a village in Mexico I have seen what happens when social security arrives. For a generation people continue in their traditional beliefs; they know how to deal with death, dying, and grief.[59] The new nurse and the doctor, thinking they know better, teach them about an evil pantheon of clinical deaths, each one of which can be banned, at a price. Instead of modernizing people's skills for self-care, they preach the ideal of hospital death. By their ministration they urge the peasants to an unending search for the good death of international description, a search that will keep them consumers forever.

---

[58] Edgar Morin, *L'Homme et la mort* (Paris: Seuil, 1970), develops the argument.

[59] Dora Ocampo, "Cuando la tristeza se mezcla con la alegría," manuscript, Mexico, November 1974.

Like all other major rituals of industrial society, medicine in practice takes the form of a game. The chief function of the physician becomes that of an umpire. He is the agent or representative of the social body, with the duty to make sure that everyone plays the game according to the rules.[60] The rules, of course, forbid leaving the game and dying in any fashion that has not been specified by the umpire. Death no longer occurs except as the self-fulfilling prophecy of the medicine man.[61]

Through the medicalization of death, health care has become a monolithic world religion[62] whose tenets

---

[60]Industrialized humanity needs therapy from crib to terminal ward. A new kind of terminal therapy is suggested by Elisabeth Kubler-Ross in *On Death and Dying* (New York: Macmillan, 1969). She maintains that the dying pass through several typical stages and that appropriate treatment can ease this process for well-managed "morituri." Paul Ramsey, "The Indignity of 'Death with Dignity,'" *Hastings Center Studies* 2 (May 1974): 47–62. There is a growing agreement among moralists in the early 1970s that death has again to be accepted and all that can be done for the dying is to keep them company in their final moments. But beneath this accord there is an increasingly mundane, naturalistic, and antihumanistic interpretation of human life. Robert S. Morison, "The Last Poem: The Dignity of the Inevitable and Necessary: Commentary on Paul Ramsey," *Hastings Center Studies* 2 (May 1974): 62–6. Morison criticizes Ramsey, who suggests that anyone unable to speak as a Christian ethicist must do so as some "hypothetical common denominator."

[61]David Lester, "Voodoo Death: Some New Thoughts on an Old Phenomenon," *American Anthropologist* 74 (June 1972): 386–90.

[62]Pierre Delooz, "Who Believes in the Hereafter?" in André Godin, ed., *Death and Presence* (Brussels: Lumen Vitae Press, 1972), pp. 17–38, shows that contemporary French public speakers have effectively separated belief in God from belief in the hereafter. Paul Danblon and André Godin, "How Do People Speak of Death?" in Godin, *ibid.*, pp. 39–62. Danblon studied interviews with 60 French-speaking public figures. The cross-denominational analogies in their expressions, feelings, and attitudes towards death are much stronger than their differences due to varying religious beliefs or practices. Joseph F. Fletcher, "Antidysthanasia: The Problem of Prolonging Death," *Journal of Pastoral Care* 18 (1964): 77–84, argues against the irresponsible prolongation of life from the point of view of a hospital chaplain: "I would myself agree with Pius XII and with at least two Archbishops of Canterbury, Lang and Fisher, who have addressed themselves to this question, that the doctor's technical knowledge and his 'educated guesses' and experience should be the basis for deciding the question as to whether there is any 'reasonable hope.' That determination is outside a layman's competence. . . . But

are taught in compulsory schools and whose ethical rules are applied to a bureaucratic restructuring of the environment: sex has become a subject in the syllabus and sharing one's spoon is discouraged for the sake of hygiene. The struggle against death, which dominates the life-style of the rich, is translated by development agencies into a set of rules by which the poor of the earth shall be forced to conduct themselves.

Only a culture that evolved in highly industrialized societies could possibly have called forth the commercialization of the death-image that I have just described. In its extreme form, "natural death" is now that point at which the human organism refuses any further input of treatment. People[63] die when the electroencephalogram indicates that their brain waves have flattened out: they do not take a last breath, or die because their heart stops. Socially approved death happens when man has become useless not only as a producer but also as a consumer. It is the point at which a consumer, trained at great expense, must finally be written off as a total loss. Dying has become the ultimate form of consumer resistance.[64]

---

having determined that the condition is hopeless, I cannot agree that it is either prudent or fair to physicians as a fraternity to saddle them with the onus of alone deciding whether to let the patient go." The thesis is common. It shows how even churches support professional judgment. This practical convergence of Christian and medical practice is in stark opposition to the attitude towards death in Christian theology. Ladislaus Boros, *Mysterium mortis: Der Mensch in der letzen Entscheidung* (Freiburg: Walter, 1962); Karl Rahner, *Zur Theologie des Todes* (Freiburg: Herder, 1963).

[63]Daniel Maguire, "The Freedom to Die," *Commonweal,* August 11, 1972, pp. 423–8. By working creatively and in ways as yet unthought of, the lobby of the dying and the gravely ill could become a healing force in society. Jonas B. Robitscher, "The Right To Die: Do We Have a Right Not To Be Treated?" *Hastings Center Studies* 2 (September 1972): 11–44.

[64]Orville Brim, et al., eds., *The Dying Patient* (New York: Russell Sage, 1960). They deal first with the spectrum of technical analysis and decision-making in which health professionals engage when faced with the task of determining the circumstances under which an individual's death should occur. They provide a series of recommendations for making this engineered process "somewhat less graceless and less distasteful for the patient, his family and most

Traditionally the person best protected from death was the one whom society had condemned to die. Society felt threatened that the man on Death Row might use his tie to hang himself. Authority might be challenged if he took his life before the appointed hour. Today, the man best protected against setting the stage for his own dying is the sick person in critical condition. Society, acting through the medical system, decides when and after what indignities and mutilations he shall die.[65] The medicalization of society has brought the epoch of natural death to an end. Western man has lost the right to preside at his act of dying. Health, or the autonomous power to cope, has been expropriated down to the last breath. Technical death has won its victory over dying.[66] Mechanical death has conquered and destroyed all other deaths.

---

of all, the attending personnel." In this anthology the macabre turns into a new kind of professionally conducted obscenity. See also David Sudnow, "Dying in a Public Hospital," in *ibid.*, pp. 191–208.

[65]David Sudnow, in his study of the social organization, reports: "A nurse was observed spending two or three minutes trying to close the eyelids of a woman patient. The nurse explained that the woman was dying. She was trying to get the lids to remain in a closed position. After several unsuccessful attempts, the nurse got them shut and said, with a sigh of accomplishment, 'Now they're right.' When questioned about what she was doing, she said that a patient's eyes must be closed after death, so that the body will resemble a sleeping person. It was more difficult to accomplish this, she explained, after the muscles and skin had begun to stiffen. She always tried, she said, to close them *before* death. This made for greater efficiency when it came time for ward personnel to wrap the body. It was a matter of consideration towards those workers who preferred to handle dead bodies as little as possible" (*ibid.*, pp. 192–3).

[66]Brillat-Savarin, "Méditation XXVI, de la mort," in *Physiologie du gout*. Brillat-Savarin attended his 93-year-old great-aunt when she was dying. "She had kept all her faculties and one would not have noticed her state but for her smaller appetite and her feeble voice. 'Are you there, nephew?' 'Yes aunt, I am at your service and I think it would be a good idea if you had some of this lovely old wine.' 'Give it to me, my friend, liquids always go down.' I made her swallow half a glass of my best wine. She perked up immediately and turning her once beautiful eyes towards me, she said, 'Thank you for this last favor. If you ever get to my age you will see that death becomes as necessary as sleep.' These were her last words and half an hour later she was asleep forever."

Part IV

The Politics of Health

6

Specific Counterproductivity

Iatrogenesis will be controlled only if it is understood as but one aspect of the destructive dominance of industry over society, as but one instance of that paradoxical counterproductivity which is now surfacing in all major industrial sectors. Like time-consuming acceleration, stupefying education, self-destructive military defense, disorienting information, or unsettling housing projects, pathogenic medicine is the result of industrial overproduction that paralyzes autonomous action. In order to focus on this specific counterproductivity of contemporary industry, frustrating overproduction must be clearly distinguished from two other categories of economic burdens with which it is generally confused, namely, declining marginal utility and negative externality. Without this distinction of the specific frustration that constitutes counterproductivity from rising prices and oppressive social costs, the social assessment of any technical enterprise, be it medicine, transportation, the media, or education, will remain limited to an accounting of cost-efficiency and not even approach a radical critique of the instrumental effectiveness of these various sectors.

Marginal Disutilities

Direct costs reflect rental charges, payments made for labor, materials, and other considerations. The production cost of a passenger-mile includes the payments made to build and operate the vehicle and the road, as well as the profit that accrues to those who have obtained control over transportation: the interest charged by the capitalists who own the tools of production, and the perquisites claimed by the bureaucrats who monopolize the stock of knowledge that is applied in the process. The price is the sum of these various rentals, no matter whether it is paid by the consumer out of his own pocket or by a tax-supported social agency that purchases on his behalf.

Negative externality is the name of the social costs that are not included in the monetary price; it is the common designation for the burdens, privations, nuisances, and injuries that I impose on others by each passenger-mile I travel. The dirt, the noise, and the ugliness my car adds to the city; the harm caused by collisions and pollution; the degradation of the total environment by the oxygen I burn and the poisons I scatter; the increasing costliness of the police department; and also the traffic-related discrimination against the poor: all are negative externalities associated with each passenger-mile. Some can easily be *internalized* in the purchase price, as for instance the damages done by collisions, which are paid for by insurance. Other externalities that do not now show up in the market price could be internalized in the same way: the cost of therapy for cancer caused by exhaust fumes could be added to each gallon of fuel, to be spent for cancer detection and surgery or for cancer prevention through antipollution devices and gas masks. But most externalities cannot be quantified and internalized: if gasoline prices are raised to reduce depletion of oil stocks and of atmospheric oxygen, each passenger-mile becomes more costly and more of a privilege; environmental damage is lessened but social injustice is increased. Beyond a certain level of intensity of industrial production, externalities cannot be reduced but only shifted around.

Counterproductivity is something other than either an individual or a social cost; it is distinct from the declining utility obtained for a unit of currency and from all forms of external disservice. It exists whenever the use of an institution paradoxically takes away from society those things the institution was designed to provide. It is a form of built-in social frustration. The price of a commodity or a service measures what the purchaser is willing to spend for whatever he gets; externalities indicate what society will tolerate to allow for this consumption; counterproductivity gauges the degree of prevalent cognitive dissonance resulting from the transaction: it is a social indicator for the built-in counterpurposive functioning of an economic sector. The iatrogenic intensity of our medical enterprise is only a particularly painful example of how frustrating overproduction appears in equal measure as time-consuming acceleration of traffic, static in communications, training for well-rounded incompetence in education, uprooting as a result of housing development, and destructive overfeeding. This specific counterproductivity constitutes an unwanted side-effect of industrial production which cannot be externalized from the particular economic sector that produces it. Fundamentally it is due neither to technical mistakes nor to class exploitation but to industrially generated destruction of those environmental, social, and psychological conditions needed for the development of nonindustrial or nonprofessional use-values. Counterproductivity is the result of an industrially induced paralysis of practical self-governing activity.

Commodities vs. Use Values

The industrial distortion of our shared perception of reality has rendered us blind to the counterpurposive level of our enterprise. We live in an epoch in which learning is planned, residence standardized, traffic motorized, and communication programmed, and in which, for the first time, a large part of all foodstuffs consumed by humanity passes through interregional markets. In such an intensely industrialized society, people are conditioned *to get* things rather than *to do* them; they are trained to value what can be purchased rather than what they themselves can create. They want to be taught, moved, treated, or guided rather than to learn, to heal, and to find their own way. Impersonal institutions are assigned personal functions. Healing ceases to be considered a task for the sick. It first becomes the duty of the individual body repairmen, and then soon changes from a personal service into the output of an anonymous agency. In the process, society is rearranged for the sake of the health-care system, and it becomes increasingly difficult to care for one's own health. Goods and services litter the domains of freedom.

Schools produce education, motor vehicles produce locomotion, and medicine produces health care. These outputs are staples that have all the characteristics of commodities. Their production costs can be added to or subtracted from the GNP, their scarcity can be measured in terms of marginal value, and their costs can be established in currency equivalents. By their very nature these staples create a market. Like school education and motor transportation, clinical care is the result of a capital-intensive commodity production; the services produced are designed for others, not with others nor for the producer.

Owing to the industrialization of our world-view, it is often overlooked that each of these commodities still competes with a nonmarketable use-value that people freely produce, each on his own. People learn by seeing and doing, they move on their feet, they heal, they take care of their health, and they contribute to the health of others. These activities have use-values that resist marketing. Most valuable learning, body movement, and healing do not show up on the

GNP. People learn their mother tongue, move around, produce their children and bring them up, recover the use of broken bones, and prepare the local diet, and do these things with more or less competence and enjoyment. These are all valuable activities which most of the time will not and cannot be undertaken for money, but which can be devalued if too much money is around.

The achievement of a concrete social goal cannot be measured in terms of industrial outputs, neither in their amount nor in the curve that represents their distribution and their social costs. The effectiveness of each industrial sector is determined by the correlation between the production of commodities by society and the autonomous production of corresponding use-values. How effective a society is in producing high levels of mobility, housing, or nutrition depends on the meshing of marketed staples with inalienable, spontaneous action.

When most needs of most people are satisfied in a domestic or community mode of production, the gap between expectation and gratification tends to be narrow and stable. Learning, locomotion, or sick-care are the results of highly decentralized initiatives, of autonomous inputs and self-limiting total outputs. Under the conditions of a subsistence economy, the tools used in production determine the needs that the application of these same tools can fulfill. For instance, people know what they can expect when they get sick. Somebody in the village or the nearby town will know all the remedies that have worked in the past, and beyond this lies the unpredictable realm of the miracle. Until late in the nineteenth century, most families, even in Western countries, provided most of the therapy that was known. Most learning, locomotion, or healing was performed by each man on his own, and the tools needed were produced in his family or village setting.

Autonomous production can, of course, be supplemented by industrial outputs that will have to be designed and often manufactured beyond direct community control. Autonomous activity can be rendered both more effective and more decentralized by using such industrially made tools as bicycles, printing presses, recorders, or X-ray equipment. But it can also be hampered, devalued, and blocked by an arrangement of society that is totally in favor of industry. The synergy between the autonomous and the heteronomous modes of production then takes on a negative cast. The arrangement of society in favor of managed commodity production has two ultimately destructive aspects: people are trained for consumption rather than for action, and at the same time their range of action is narrowed. The tool separates the workman from his labor. Habitual bicycle commuters are pushed off the road by intolerable levels of traffic, and patients accustomed to taking care of their own ailments find yesterday's remedies available only on prescription and hence largely unobtainable. Wage labor and client relationships expand while autonomous production and gift relationships wither.

Effectively achieving social objectives depends on the degree to which the two fundamental modes of production supplement or hamper each other. Effectively coming to know and to control a given physical and social environment depends on people's formal education and on their opportunity and motivation to learn in a nonprogrammed way. Effective traffic depends on the ability of people to get where they must go quickly and conveniently. Effective sick-care depends on the degree to which pain and dysfunction are made tolerable and recovery is enhanced. The effective satisfaction of these needs must be clearly distinguished from the efficiency with which industrial products are made and marketed, from the number of certificates, passenger-miles, housing units, or medical interventions performed. Beyond a certain threshold, these outputs will all be needed only as remedies; they will substitute for personal activities that previous industrial outputs have paralyzed. The social criteria by which effective need-satisfaction can be evaluated do not match the measurements used to evaluate the production and marketing of industrial goods.

Since measurements disregard the contributions made by the autonomous mode towards the total effectiveness with which any major social goal may be achieved, they cannot indicate if this total effectiveness is increasing or decreasing. The number of graduates, for instance, might be inversely related to general competence. Much less can technical measurements indicate who are the beneficiaries and who are the losers from industrial growth, who are the few that get more and can do more and who fall into the majority whose marginal access to industrial products is compounded by their loss of autonomous effectiveness. Only political judgment can assess the balance.

Modernization of Poverty

The persons most hurt by counterproductive institutionalization are usually not the poorest in monetary terms. The typical victims of the depersonalization of values are the powerless in a milieu made for the industrially enriched. Among the powerless may be people who are relatively affluent within their society or those who are inmates of benevolent total institutions. Disabling dependence reduces them to modernized poverty. Policies meant to remedy the new sense of privation will not only be futile but will aggravate the damage. By promising more staples rather than protecting autonomy, they will intensify disabling dependence.

The poor in Bengal or Peru still survive with occasional employment and an occasional dip into the market economy: they live by the timeless art of making do. They still can stretch out provisions, alternate between fat and lean periods, knit gift relationships whereby they barter or otherwise exchange goods and services neither made for nor accounted for by the market. In the country, in the absence of television, they enjoy living in homes built on traditional models. Drawn or pushed into town, they squat on the margins of the steel-and-petroleum sector, where they build a provisional economy with scraps of waste that can serve as building blocks for self-made shacks. Their exposure to extreme famine grows with their dependence on marketed food.

Given sufficient generations, during its entire evolution *Homo sapiens* has shown high competence in developing a great variety of cultural forms, each meant to keep the total population of a region within the limits of resources that could be shared or formally exchanged in its bounded milieu. The worldwide and homogeneous disabling of the communal coping ability of local populations has developed with imperialism and its contemporary variants of industrial development and compassionate chic.

The invasion of the underdeveloped countries by new instruments of production organized for financial efficiency rather than local effectiveness and for professional rather than lay control inevitably disqualifies tradition and autonomous learning and creates the need for therapy from teachers, doctors, and social workers. While road and radio mold the lives of those whom they reach to industrial standards, they degrade their handicrafts, housing, or health care much faster than they crush the skills they replace. Aztec massage gives relief to many who would no longer admit it because they believe it outdated. The common family bed becomes disreputable much faster than its occupants become aware of discomfort. Where development plans have worked, they have often succeeded because of the unforeseen resilience of the adobe-cum-oildrum sector. The continued ability to produce foods on marginal land and in city backyards has saved productivity campaigns from the Ukraine to Venezuela. The ability to care for the sick, the old, and the insane without nurses or wardens has buffered the majority against the rising specific disutilities which symbolic enrichment has brought. Poverty in the subsistence sector, even when this subsistence is retrenched by considerable market dependence, does not crush autonomy. People remain motivated to squat on thoroughfares, to nibble at professional monopolies, or to circumvent the bureaucrats.

When perception of personal needs is the result of professional diagnosis, dependence turns into painful disability. The aged in the United States can again serve as the paradigm. They have been trained to experience urgent needs that no level of *relative* privilege can possibly satisfy. The more tax money that is spent to bolster their fraility, the keener is their awareness of decay. At the same time, their ability to take care of themselves has withered, as social arrangements allowing them to exercise autonomy have practically disappeared. The aged are an example of the specialization of poverty which the over-specialization of services can bring forth. The elderly in the United States are only one extreme example of suffering promoted by high-cost deprivation. Having learned to consider old age akin to disease, they have developed unlimited economic needs in order to pay for interminable therapies, which are usually ineffective, are frequently demeaning and painful, and call more often than not for reclusion in a special milieu.

Five faces of industrially modernized poverty appear caricatured in the pampered ghettos of rich men's retirement: the incidence of chronic disease increases as fewer people die in their youth; more people suffer clinical damage from health measures; medical services grow more slowly than the spread and urgency of demand; people find fewer resources in their environment and culture to help them come to terms with their suffering, and thus are forced to depend on medical services for a wider range of trivia; people lose the ability to live with impairment or pain and become dependent on the management of every discomfort by specialized service personnel. The cumulative result of overexpansion in the health-care industry has thwarted the power of people to respond to challenges and to cope with changes in their bodies or their environment.

The destructive power of medical overexpansion does not, of course, mean that sanitation, inoculation, and vector control, well-distributed health education, healthy architecture, and safe machinery, general competence in first aid, equally distributed access to dental and primary medical care, as well as judiciously selected complex services, could not all fit into a truly modern culture that fostered self-care and autonomy. As long as engineered intervention in the relationship between individuals and environment remains below a certain intensity, relative to the range of the individual's freedom of action, such intervention could enhance the organism's competence in coping and creating its own future. But beyond a certain level, the heteronomous management of life will inevitably first restrict, then cripple, and finally paralyze the organism's nontrivial responses, and what was meant to constitute health care will turn into a specific form of health denial.[1]

---

[1]About pathogenic role-assignment, particularly in contemporary industrial society, see H. P. Dreitzel, *Die gesellschaftlichen Leiden und das Leiden an der Gesellschaft: Vorstudien zu einer Pathologie des Rollenverhaltens* (Stuttgart: Enke, 1972).

7

Political Countermeasures

Fifteen years ago it would have been impossible to get a hearing for the claim that medicine itself might be a danger to health. In the early 1960s, the British National Health Service still enjoyed a worldwide reputation, particularly among American reformers.[1] The service, created by Albert Beveridge, was based on the assumption that there exists in every population a strictly limited amount of morbidity which, if treated under conditions of equity, will eventually decline.[2] Thus Beveridge had calculated

---

[1]Charles E. A. Winslow, *The Cost of Sickness and the Price of Health* (Geneva: World Health Organization, 1951). Daniel S. Hirshfield, *The Lost Reform: The Campaign for Compulsory Health Insurance in the United States from 1932 to 1943* (Cambridge, Mass.: Harvard Univ. Press, 1970), describes the failure so far of the uninsured minority of the aged, poor, and chronically ill to muster support for protective laws from the largely contented majority. He shows that the earlier problems, attitudes towards them, and approaches remain largely unchanged in the 1970s. It seems that at no time has public-policy discussion of health care transcended the industrial paradigm of medicine as a biological and social enterprise.

[2]For a history of welfare legislation see Henry E. Sigerist, "From Bismarck to Beveridge: Developments and Trends in Social Security

that the annual cost of the Health Service would fall as therapy reduced the rate of illness.[3] Health planners and welfare economists never expected that the service's redefinition of health would broaden the scope of medical care and that only budgetary restrictions would keep it from expanding indefinitely. It was not predicted that soon, in a regional screening, only sixty-seven out of one thousand people would be found completely fit and that 50 percent would be referred to a doctor, while according to another study, one in six people screened would be defined as suffering from one to nine serious illnesses.[4] Nor had the health planners forecast that the threshold of tolerance for everyday reality would decline as fast as the competence for self-care was undermined, and that one-quarter of all visits to the doctor for free service would be for the untreatable common cold. Between 1943 and 1951, 75 percent of the persons questioned claimed to have suffered from illness during the preceding month.[5] By 1972, 95 percent of those surveyed in one study considered themselves unwell during the fourteen days prior to questioning, and in another study[6] in which 5 percent considered

---

Legislation," *Bulletin of the History of Medicine* 13 (April 1943): 365–88. For a rather naïvely enthusiastic evaluation of analogous legislation in Russia, see Henry E. Sigerist, *Socialized Medicine in the Soviet Union* (1937; rev. ed., as *Medicine and Health in the Soviet Union,* New York: Citadel Press, 1947).

[3]Office of Health Economics, *Prospects in Health,* Publication no. 37 (London, 1971).

[4]R. G. S. Brown, *The Changing National Health Service* (London: Routledge, 1973), and S. Israel and G. Teeling Smith, "The Submerged Iceberg of Sickness in Society," *Social and Economic Administration,* vol. 1, no. 1 (1967). For every case of diabetes, rheumatism, or epilepsy known to the general practitioner, there appears to be another case undiagnosed. For each known case of psychiatric illness, bronchitis, high blood pressure, glaucoma, or urinary-tract infection, there are likely to be five cases undiscovered. The cases of untreated anemia probably exceed those treated eightfold.

[5]W. P. D. Logan and E. Brooke, *Survey of Sickness, 1943–51* (London: Her Majesty's Stationery Office, 1957).

[6]Karen Dunnell and Ann Cartwright, *Medicine Takers, Prescribers and Hoarders* (London: Routledge, 1972).

themselves free of symptoms, 9 percent claimed to have suffered from more than six different symptoms in the two weeks just past. Least of all did the health planners make provision for the new diseases that would become endemic through the same process that made medicine at least partially effective.[7] They did not forecast the need for special hospitals dedicated to the soothing of terminal pain, usually suffered by the victims of unsound or ineffective surgery for cancer,[8] or the need for other hospital beds for those affected by medicine-induced disease.[9]

The sixties also witnessed the rise and fall of a multinational consortium for the export of optimism to the third world which took shape in the Peace Corps, the Alliance for Progress, Israeli aid to Central Africa, and in the last brush-fires of medical-missionary zeal. The Western belief that its medicines could cure the ills of the nonindustrialized tropics was then at its height. International cooperation had just won major battles against mosquitoes, microbes, and parasites, ultimately Pyrrhic victories which were advertised as the beginning of a final solution to tropical disease.[10] The role that economic and technological development would play in spreading and aggravating sleeping sickness, bilharziasis, and even ma-

---

[7]This was the period of mass screening for disorders that educators, economists, or physicians could detect. It was still considered "progress" when tests conducted on 1,709 people revealed more than 90% to be suffering from some disease. J. E. Shental, "Multiphasic Screening of the Well Patient," *Journal of the American Medical Association* 172 (1960): 1–4.

[8]Frank Turnbull, "Pain and Suffering in Cancer," *Canadian Nurse*, August 1971, pp. 28–31. Turnbull argues that though surgical or radiological treatment may cause a recession in the primary symptoms that might have led to a painless death, it may also allow development of secondary disease that is more painful.

[9]Estimated at 12–18% of all U.S. hospital beds.

[10]M. Taghi Farvar and John P. Milton, eds., *The Careless Technology* (Garden City, N.Y.: Natural History Press, 1972). Scientific papers from a conference held in 1968, indicating that the post-World War II idea that traditional societies can and should be overhauled overnight has proved not only virtually unachievable but also undesirable in view of the serious consequences for man's organism.

laria was not yet suspected.[11] Those who saw world hunger and new pestilence on the horizon were treated like prophets of doom[12] or romantics;[13] the Green Revolution was still considered the opening phase of a healthier and more equitable world.[14] It

---

[11]Charles C. Hughes and John M. Hunter, "Disease and Development in Africa," *Social Science and Medicine* 3, no. 4 (1970): 443–88. An important survey of the literature on disease consequences of developmental activities. Ralph J. Audy, "Aspects of Human Behavior Interfering with Vector Control," in *Vector Control and the Recrudesence of Vector-borne Diseases,* Proceedings of a Symposium Held During the Tenth Meeting of the PAHO Advisory Committee on Medical Research, June 15, 1971, Pan-American Health Organization Scientific Publication no. 238 (Washington, D.C., 1972), pp. 67–82.

[12]René Dumont, *La Faim du monde,* complete text of a conference held in Liège November 8, 1965, followed by responses to the 25 questions discussed (Liége/Brussels: Cercle d'Éducation Populaire, 1966). An impassioned appeal for world solidarity at the eleventh hour. A later English version is René Dumont and Bernard Rosier, *The Hungry Future* (New York: Praeger, 1969). For a right-wing complement to this view from the left, consult William and Paul Paddock, *Famine Nineteen Seventy-five! America's Decision: Who Will Survive?* (Boston: Little, Brown, 1967). Early debunkers of the dreams of their decade, such as hydroponics, desalinization, synthetic foods, and ocean farming, the authors are also convinced that land reform, irrigation, and fertilizer production cannot avert famine. They foresee increased dependence of the world on U.S. outputs, and propose "triage," i.e., selection, by the U.S. of those to be kept alive.

[13]Marshall Sahlins, *Stone Age Economics* (Chicago: Aldine-Atherton, 1972), points out that the institutionalized hunger of the 1960s is an unprecedented phenomenon, and accumulates evidence that in a typical Stone Age culture a much smaller percentage of people than today went to bed malnourished and hungry.

[14]George Borgstrom, "The Green Revolution," in *Focal Points* (New York: Macmillan, 1972), pt. 2, pp. 172–201. An analysis and appraisal of a dozen illusions about the Green Revolution, many of which are constantly reinforced by misleading statements from international agencies. On the dangers of genetic depletion, consult National Academy of Sciences, *Genetic Vulnerability of Major Crops* (Washington, D.C., 1972). Since paleolithic times, each human society has developed a rich variety of cereals and other food crops. The strains that have survived are those favored by populations fed largely on grains and legumes. Although inferior in yield per acre to engineered hybrids, these strains are adaptable, are independent of fertilizers, irrigation, and pest control, and have a high potential for future adaptation. Entire populations of such rich genetic mixtures have been wiped out by replacement with hybrids. The damage done in a ten-year period is irreparable and of unforeseeable consequences.

would have seemed unbelievable that within ten years *malnutrition* in two forms would become by far the most important threat to modern man.[15] The new high-caloric undernourishment of poor populations was not foreseen,[16] nor was the fact that overfeeding would be identified as the main cause for the epidemic diseases of the rich.[17] In the United States the new frontiers had not yet been obstructed by competing bureaucratic schemes.[18] Hopes for better health still focused on equality of access to the agencies that would do away with specific diseases. Iatrogenesis was still an issue for the paranoid.

But by 1975 much of this had changed.[19] A generation ago, children in kindergarten had painted the doctor as a white-coated father-figure.[20] Today,

---

[15]For an introduction to the state of discussion on world nutrition, see Alan Berg, *The Nutrition Factor: Its Role in National Development* (Washington, D.C.: Brookings Institution, 1973). The valuable bibliography must be mined out of the footnotes. See also J. Hemardinquer, "Pour une histoire de l'alimentation," *Cahiers des Annales* 28 (Paris: Colin, 1970).

[16]On one consequence of exporting Dr. Spock to the tropics, see A. E. Davis and T. D. Bolin, "Lactose Tolerance in Southeast Asia," in Farvar and Milton, eds., *The Careless Technology.*

[17]Adelle Davis, *Let's Eat Right To Keep Fit* (New York: Harcourt Brace, 1970). A well-documented report on the qualitative decline of U.S. diet with the rise of industrialization and on the reflection of this decline in U.S. health.

[18]For orientation on the controversy, consult Edward M. Kennedy, *In Critical Condition: The Crisis in America's Health Care* (New York: Pocket Books, 1973). For a summary of the controversy, see Stephen Jonas, "Issues in National Health Insurance in the United States of America," *Lancet,* 1974, 2:143–6, William R. Roy, *The Proposed Health Maintenance Organization Act of 1972,* Science and Health Communications Group Sourcebook Series, vol. 2 (Washington, D.C., 1972). A Kansas congressman explains and defends the bill he introduced in Congress and marshals concurring opinion.

[19]An excellent, if now dated, forecast is Michael Michaelson, "The Coming Medical War," *New York Review of Books,* July 1, 1971. See also Robert Bremner, *From the Depths: The Discovery of Poverty in the U.S.* (New York: New York Univ. Press, 1956), an introduction to the origins of the U.S. social welfare movement.

[20]Barbara Myerhoff and William R. Larson, "The Doctor as Cultural Hero: The Routinization of Charisma," *Human Organization* 24 (fall 1965): 188–91. The authors predicted that the doctor would soon appear in an increasingly prosaic light, thus losing the psychological power he traditionally had to gain the patient's confidence and to act as a healer.

however, they will just as readily paint him as a man from Mars or a Frankenstein.[21] Muckracking feeds on medical charts and doctors' tax returns, and a new mood of wariness among patients has caused medical and pharmaceutical companies to triple their expenses for public relations.[22] Ralph Nader has made the consumers of health staples money- and quality-conscious. The ecological movement has created an awareness that health depends on the environment—on food and working conditions and housing—and Americans have come to accept the idea that they are threatened by pesticides,[23] additives,[24] and mycotoxins[25] and other health risks due to environmental

---

[21]Michel Maccoby, personal communication to the author.

[22]John Pekkanen, *The American Connection: Profiteering and Politicking in the "Ethical" Drug Industry* (Chicago: Follett, 1973). A report on the willful manipulation of political power, influence, and personalities by the U.S. Pharmaceutical Manufacturers Association (PMA) and the drug lobby to maintain profits by overproducing and overselling drugs and systematically hiding hazards behind advertising, promotion, and the systematic corruption of highly placed physicians. Cites specific charges against two dozen named major firms.

[23]Paul R. and Anne H. Ehrlich, *Population, Resources, Environment: Issues in Human Ecology* (San Francisco: Freeman, 1972), particularly chap. 7 on ecosystems in jeopardy, provides a good introduction to the literature on the subject. Samuel Epstein and Marvin Legator, eds., *The Mutagenicity of Pesticides: Concepts and Evaluation* (Cambridge, Mass.: MIT Press, 1971), yields many specific data. Harrison Wellford, *Sowing the Wind: Report on the Politics of Food Safety*, Ralph Nader's Study Group Reports (New York: Grossman, 1972). A report on pesticide concentrations in food. The misuse of pesticides threatens the farmer even more than it does the city dweller; it destroys his health, raises the cost of production, and tends to lower long-term yields. J. L. Radomski, W. B. Deichman, and E. E. Clizer, "Pesticide Concentration in the Liver, Brain, and Adipose Tissue of Terminal Hospital Patients," *Food and Cosmetics Toxicology* 6 (1968): 209–20. A very frightening quantitative analysis.

[24]James S. Turner, *The Chemical Feast: A Report on the Food and Drug Administration*, Ralph Nader's Study Group Reports (New York: Grossman, 1970). This report indicates that the trend described by Adelle Davis in *Let's Eat Right to Keep Fit* is accelerating and that the damage done to health by bad nutrition increased during the 1960's. It points out that less than half the more than 2,000 food additives in use have been tested for safety.

[25]Arturo Aldama, "Los cereales envenenados: Otra enfermedad del progreso," CIDOC Document I/V 74/58, Cuernavaca, 1974.

degradation. Women's liberation has highlighted the key role that the control over one's body plays in health care.[26] A few slum communities have assumed responsibility for basic health care and have tried to unhook their members from dependence on outsiders. The class-specific nature of body perception,[27] language,[28] concepts,[29] access to health services,[30] infant mortality,[31] and actual, specifically chronic, morbidity[32] has been widely documented, and the class-

---

[26]Boston Women's Health Collective, *Our Bodies, Ourselves: A Book By and For Women* (New York: Simon & Schuster, 1973). Can be considered a model guide for limited self-care elaborated by a group of women who remain deeply committed to a basically medicalized society.

[27]Luc Boltanski, *Consommation médicale et rapport au corps: Compte-rendu de fin de contrat d'une recherche financée par la Délégation Générale à la Recherche Scientifique et Technique* (Paris: Centre de Sociologie Européenne, 1969). A sociology of the body: a pioneer study of the social determinants of the individual's relationship to his own body depending on his social class.

[28]See Liselotte von Ferber, "Die Diagnose des praktischen Arztes in Spiegel der Patientenangaben," in *Schriftenreihe: Arbeitsmedizin, Sozialmedizin, Arbeitshygiene,* vol. 43 (Stuttgart: Gentner, 1971), on the class-specific language in German general practice.

[29]Charles Kadushin, "Social Class and the Experience of Ill Health," *Sociological Inquiry* 34 (1964): 67–80, challenges the sociological dogma of an association between socio-economic status and the occurrence of chronic disease. David Mechanic, *Medical Sociology: A Selective View* (New York: Free Press, 1968), pp. 259 ff., provides contradictory arguments and literature; see also p. 245 on infant mortality, p. 253 on socio-economic status.

[30]Raymond S. Duff and August B. Hollingshead, *Sickness and Society* (New York: Harper & Row, 1961). S. H. King, *Perceptions of Illness and Medical Practice* (New York: Russell Sage, 1962).

[31]Mechanic, *Medical Sociology*. See especially pp. 267–8 as an introduction to the U.S. National Health Service statistics on socio-economic status and the use of health services. Beware of taking these data at face value: see David Mechanic and M. Newton, "Some Problems in the Analysis of Morbidity Data," *Journal of Chronic Diseases* 18 (June 1965): 569–80. Lee Rainwater and W. L. Yancey, *The Moynihan Report and the Politics of Controversy* (Cambridge, Mass.: MIT Press, 1967), discuss the complexity of associations between infant mortality and socio-economic deprivation.

[32]Barbara Blackwell, *The Literature of Delay in Seeking Medical Care for Chronic Illnesses,* Health Education Monograph no. 16 (San Francisco: Society for Public Health Education, 1963). See especially pp. 14–17 for delay related to personal, physical, and social attributes. René Lenoir, *Les Exclus* (Paris: Seuil, 1974), focuses attention on the institutional creation of needy dropouts from various health-care systems in France.

specific origins[33] and prejudices[34] of physicians are beginning to be understood. The World Health Organization, meanwhile, is moving to a conclusion that would have shocked most of its founders: in a recent publication WHO advocates the deprofessionalization of primary care as the most important single step in raising national health levels.[35]

Doctors themselves are beginning to look askance at what doctors do.[36] When physicians in New England were asked to evaluate the treatment their patients had received from other doctors, most were dissatisfied. Depending on the method of peer evaluation used, between 1.4 percent and 63 percent of patients were believed to have received *adequate* care.[37] Patients are told ever more frequently by their

---

[33]G. Kleinbach, "Social Class and Medical Education," thesis, Department of Education, Harvard University, 1974. Charles F. Schumacher, "The 1960 Medical School Graduate: His Biographical History," *Journal of Medical Education* 36 (1961): 401 ff., shows that more than half of medical students are children of professionals or managers.

[34]Howard Becker et al., *Boys in White: Student Culture in Medical School* (1961: reprint ed., Dubuque, Iowa: William C. Brown, 1972).

[35]Kenneth W. Newell, ed., *Health by the People* (Geneva: World Health Organization, 1975). V. Djukanovic, and E. P. Mach, Alternative approaches to meeting basic health needs in developing countries. A joint UNICEF/WHO study. Geneva, World Health Organization, 1975. "Some aspects of what may be called conventional health services are singled out as factors in the failure of the present systems to meet the basic health needs in developing countries."

[36]On the emergence of social medicine as a discipline, see first Thomas McKeon and C. R. Lowe, *An Introduction to Social Medicine* (Oxford/Edinburgh: Blackwell Scientific Publications, 1966), pp. ix–xiii. Then see Gordon McLachlan, ed., *Portfolio for Health* 2 (New York/Toronto: Nuffield Provincial Hospitals Trust and Oxford University Press, 1973). For the German literature in the field see Hans Schaefer and Maria Blohmke, *Sozialmedizin: Einführung in die Ergebnisse und Probleme der Medizin-Soziologie und Sozialmedizin* (Stuttgart: Thieme, 1972). For Eastern Europe see Richard E. and Shirley B. Weinerman, *Social Medicine in Eastern Europe: The Organization of Health Services and the Education of the Medical Personnel in Czechoslovakia, Hungary and Poland* (Cambridge, Mass.: Harvard University Press, 1969). For Italy, see Giovanni Berlinguer, *Medicina e politica* (Bari: De Donato, 1976).

[37]Robert H. Brook and Francis A. Appel, "Quality-of-Care Assessment: Choosing a Method for Peer Review," *New England Journal of Medicine* 288 (1973): 1323–9. Judgments based on group

doctors that they have been damaged by previous medication and that the treatment now prescribed is made necessary by the effects of such prior medication, which in some cases was given in a life-saving endeavor, but much more often for weight control, mild hypertension, flu, or mosquito bite or just to put a mutually satisfactory conclusion to an interview with the doctor.[38] In 1973 a retiring senior official of the U.S. Department of Health, Education, and Welfare could say that 80 percent of all funds channeled through his office provided no demonstrable benefits to health and that much of the rest was spent to offset iatrogenic damage. His successor will have to deal with these data if he wants to maintain public trust.[39]

Patients are starting to listen, and a growing number of movements and organizations are beginning to demand reform. The attacks are founded on five major categories of criticism and are directed to five categories of reform: (1) Production of remedies and services has become self-serving. Consumer lobbies and consumer control of hospital boards should therefore force doctors to improve their wares. (2) The delivery of remedies and access to services is unequal and arbitrary; it depends either on the patient's money and rank, or on social and medical prejudices which favor, for example, attention to heart disease over attention to malnutrition. The nationalization of health production ought to control the hidden biases of the clinic. (3) The organization of the medical

---

consensus, as opposed to the criteria selected by individual reviewers, yielded the fewest acceptable cases. Robert H. Brook and Robert Stevenson, Jr., "Effectiveness of Patient Care in an Emergency Room," *New England Journal of Medicine* 283 (1970): 904–6.

[38]Jean-Pierre Dupuy, "Le Médicament dans la relation médecin-malade," *Projet*, no. 75 (May 1973), pp. 532–46.

[39]Arnold I. Kisch and Leo G. Reeder, "Client Evaluation of Physician Performance," *Journal of Health and Social Behavior* 10 (1969): 51–8. While it is generally assumed that quality control in professional service must depend on self-policing—bad as this might be—the results of a study conducted in Los Angeles indicate that patients' rating of physican performance closely corresponded with a number of criteria of quality in medical care generally accepted as valid by health professionals.

guild perpetuates inefficiency and privilege, while professional licensing of specialists fosters an increasingly narrow and specialized view of disease. A combination of capitation payment with institutional licensing ought to combine control over doctors with the interest of patients. (4) The sway of one kind of medicine deprives society of the benefits competing sects might offer. More public support for alpha waves, encounter groups, and chiropractic ought to countervail and complement the scalpel and the poison. (5) The main thrust of present medicine is the individual, in sickness or in health. More resources for the engineering of populations and environments ought to stretch the health dollar.

These proposed remedial policies could control to some degree the social costs created by overmedicalization. By joining together, consumers do have power to get more for their money: welfare bureaucracies do have the power to reduce inequalities; changes in licensing and in modes of financing can protect the population not only against nonprofessional quacks but also, in some cases, against professional abuse; money transferred from the production of human spare parts to the reduction of industrial risks does buy more "health" per dollar. But all these policies, unless carefully qualified, will tend to reduce the *externalities* created by medicine at the cost of a further increase of medicine's paradoxical counterproduct, its negative effect on health. All tend to stimulate further medicalization. All consistently place the improvement of medical services above those factors which would improve and equalize opportunities, competence, and confidence for self-care; they deny the civil liberty to live and to heal, and substitute promises of more conspicuous social entitlements to care by a professional.

In the following five sections I will deal with some of these possible countermeasures and examine their relative merits.

Consumer Protection for Addicts

When people become aware of their dependence on the medical industry, they tend to be trapped in the belief that they are already hopelessly hooked. They fear a life of disease without a doctor much as they would feel immobilized without a car or a bus. In this state of mind they are ready to be organized for consumer protection and to seek solace from politicians who will check the high-handedness of medical producers.[40] The need for such self-protection is obvious, the implicit dangers obscure. The sad truth for consumer advocates is that neither control of cost nor assurance of quality guarantees that health will be served by medicine that measures up to present medical standards.

Consumers who band together to force General Motors to produce an acceptable car have begun to feel competent to look under the hood and to develop criteria for estimating the cost of a cleaner exhaust system. When they band together for better health care, they still believe—mistakenly—that they are unqualified to decide what ought to be done for their bowels and kidneys and blindly entrust themselves to the doctor for almost any repair. Cross-cultural comparison of practices provides no guide. Prescriptions for vitamins are seven times more common in Britain than in Sweden, gamma globulin medication eight times more common in Sweden than in Britain. American doctors operate, on the average, twice as often as Britons; French surgeons amputate almost up to the neck. Median hospital stays vary not with the affliction but with the physician: for peptic ulcers,

---

[40]For examples of public reports on research in the service of consumer advocacy in the health field, see Robert S. McCleery, *One Life—One Physician* (Washington, D.C.: Public Affairs Press, 1971); also Joseph Page and Mary-Win O'Brien, *Bitter Wages: The Report on Disease and Injury on the Job*, Ralph Nader's Study Group Reports (New York: Grossman, 1973), an indictment of industrial and occupational medicine as practiced up to 1968. Crass underreporting of injuries sustained on the job has fostered the belief that carelessness of workers is their main cause.

from six to twenty-six days; for myocardial infarction, from ten to thirty days. The average length of stay in a French hospital is twice that in the United States. Appendectomies are performed and deaths from appendicitis are diagnosed three times more frequently in Germany than anywhere else.[41]

Titmuss[42] has summed up the difficulty of cost-benefit accounting in medicine, especially at a time when medical care is losing the characteristics it used to possess when it consisted almost wholly in the personal doctor-patient relationship. Medical care is uncertain and unpredictable; many consumers do not desire it, do not know they need it, and cannot know in advance what it will cost them. They cannot learn from experience. They must rely on the supplier to tell them if they have been well served, and they cannot return the service to the seller or have it repaired. Medical services are not advertised as are other goods, and the producer discourages comparison. Once he has purchased, a consumer cannot change his mind in mid-treatment. By defining what constitutes illness the medical producer has the power to select his consumers and to market some products that will be forced on the consumer, if need be, by the intervention of the police: the producers can even sell forcible internment for the disabled and asylums for the mentally retarded. Malpractice suits have mitigated the layman's sense of impotence on several of these points,[43] but basically, they have

---

[41]For more data and references see Michael H. Cooper, *Rationing Health Care* (London: Halsted Press, 1975), and International Bank for Reconstruction and Development, *Health Sector Policy Paper,* Washington, D.C., March 1975. Note also that the average number of days spent by a patient in the hospital varies greatly among countries with comparable GNP, even when these countries are poor. In Senegal it is 24 days, in Thailand 5.8.

[42]Richard M. Titmuss, "The Culture of Medical Care and Consumer Behaviour," in F. N. L. Poynter, ed., *Medicine and Culture* (London: Wellcome Institute, 1969), chap. 8, pp. 129–35.

[43]On the impact that malpractice suits have on the patient's perception of his body as a form of capital investment, see, e.g., Nathan Hershey, "The Defensive Practice of Medicine—Myth or Reality?" *Milbank Memorial Fund Quarterly* 50 (January 1972): 69–98.

reinforced the patient's determination to insist on treatment that is considered adequate by informed *medical* opinion. What further complicates matters is that there is no "normal" consumer of medical services. Nobody knows how much health care will be worth to him in terms of money or pain. In addition, nobody knows if the most advantageous form of health care is obtained from medical producers, from a travel agent, or by renouncing work on the night shift. The family that forgoes a car to move into a Manhattan apartment can foresee how the substitution of rent for gas will affect their available time; but the person who, upon the diagnosis of cancer, chooses an operation over a binge in the Bahamas does not know what effect his choice will have on his remaining time of grace. The economics of health is a curious discipline, somewhat reminiscent of the theology of indulgences which flourished before Luther. You can count what the friars collect, you can look at the temples they build, you can take part in the liturgies they indulge in, but you can only guess what the traffic in remission from purgatory does to the soul after death. Models developed to account for the willingness of taxpayers to foot rising medical bills constitute similar scholastic guesswork about the new world-spanning church of medicine. To give an example: it is possible to view health as durable capital stock used to produce an output called "healthy time.[44] Individuals inherit an initial stock, which can be increased by investment in health capitalization through the acquisition of medical care, or through good diet and housing. "Healthy time" is an article in demand for two reasons. As a consumer commodity, it directly enters into the individual's utility function; people usually would rather be healthy than sick. It also enters the market as an investment commodity. In this function, "healthy time" determines the amount of time an individual can spend on work

---

[44]Michael Grossman, "On the Concept of Health Capital and the Demand for Health," *Journal of Political Economy* 80 (March–April 1972): 223–55.

and on play, on earning and on recreation. The individual's "healthy time" can thus be viewed as a decisive indicator of his value to the community as a producer.[45]

Orientation on policy and theories on the dollar value of "health" production divide the adherents of squabbling academic factions much as realism and nominalism divided medieval divines.[46] But to the point that concerns the consumer, they just state in a roundabout way what every Mexican bricklayer knows: only on those days when he is healthy enough to work can he bring beans and tortillas to his children and have a tequila with his friends.[47] The belief in a causal relationship between doctor's bills and health—which would otherwise be called modernized superstition—is a basic technical assumption for the medical economist.[48]

Different systems have been used to legitimize the economic value of the specific activities in which physicians engage. Socialist nations assume the financing of all care and leave it to the medical pro-

---

[45] P. E. Enterline, "Sick Absence in Certain Western Countries," *Industrial Medicine and Surgery* 33 (October 1964): 738.

[46] For orientation on the literature, consult Kathleen N. Williams, comp., *Health and Development: An Annotated Indexed Bibliography* (Baltimore: Johns Hopkins University School of Hygiene and Public Health, Department of International Health, 1972), 931 items on health, however measured, and its supposed relationship to economic development. Constructed as a working instrument for health-resources allocation, it is particularly valuable for its references and summaries of Eastern European studies.

[47] Herbert Pollack and Donald R. Sheldon, "The Factor of Disease in the World Food Problem," *Journal of the American Medical Association* 212 (1970): 598–603. Sick people burn more food per unit of work done and also produce less work. In both ways, endemic disease adds to the world food shortage.

[48] Ralph Audy, "Health as Quantifiable Property," *British Medical Journal,* 1973, 4:486–7. Audy is one of the rare authors who go beyond trivial economy and develop a model for the dimensional analysis of man in relation to his environment. He regards health as a continuing property that can potentially be measured in terms of one's ability to "rally from challenges to adapt." Speed and success in rallying depend on the amount of protection provided by a person's habitual "cocoons" and on society's "health" in general.

fession to define what is needed, how it must be done, who may do it, what it should cost, and who shall get it. More brazenly than elsewhere, input/output calculations of such investments in human capital seem to determine Russian allocations.[49] Most welfare states intervene with laws and incentives in the organization of their health-care markets, although only the United States has launched a national legislative program under which committees of producers determine what outputs offered on the "free market" the state shall approve as "good care." In late 1973 President Nixon signed Public Law 92-603 establishing mandatory cost and quality controls (by Professional Standard Review Organizations) for Medicaid and Medicare, the tax-supported sector of the health-care industry, which since 1970 has been second in size only to the military-industrial complex. Harsh financial sanctions threaten physicians who refuse to open their files to government inspectors searching for evidence of over-utilization of hospitals, fraud, or deficient treatment. The law requires the medical profession to establish guidelines for the diagnosis and treatment of a long list of injuries, illnesses, and health conditions, mandating the world's most costly program for the medicalization of health production through legislated consumer protection.[50] The new

---

[49]See Williams, *Health and Development*, chapter on Soviet medical economy.

[50]Claude Welch, "Professional Standards Review Organizations—Pros and Cons," *New England Journal of Medicine* 290 (1974): 1319 ff.; *idem,* 289 (1973): 291–5. David E. Willett, "PSRO Today: A Lawyer's Assessment," *New England Journal of Medicine* 292 (1975): 340–3; see also editorial about this article in same number, p. 365. Victor W. Sidel, "Quality for whom?" Effects of professional responsibility for quality of health care on equity in: Bulletin of the New York Academy of Medicine. Second series, vol. 52, No. 1, January, 1976. pp. 164–176. When professionals are not limited to the role of mere technical consultants in the process of quality control, quality in health-care will be (1) defined as an enhancement of the professionals' self-image (2) as an applicator of technical factors (3) encompassing technology rather than equity and (4) will be harmful to health as perceived by the community. An important outline!

law guarantees the standard set by *industry* for the commodity. It *does not* ask if its delivery is positively or negatively related to the health of people.

Attempts to exercise rational political control over the production of medical health care have consistently failed. The reason lies in the nature of the product now called "medicine," a package made up of chemicals, apparatus, buildings, and specialists, and delivered to the client. The purveyor rather than his clients or political boss determines the size of the package. The patient is reduced to an object—his body—being repaired; he is no longer a subject being helped to heal. If he is allowed to participate in the repair process, he acts as the lowest apprentice in a hierarchy of repairmen.[51] Often he is not even trusted to take a pill without the supervision of a nurse.

The argument that institutional health care (remedial or preventive) ceases after a certain point to correlate with any further "gains" in health can be misused for transforming clients hooked on doctors into clients of some other service hegemony: nursing homes, social workers, vocational counselors, schools.[52] What started out as a defense of consumers against inadequate medical service, will, first, provide the medical profession with assurance of continued demand and then with the power to delegate some of these services to other industrial branches: to the producers of foods, mattresses, vacations, or training. Consumer protection thus turns quickly into a crusade to transform independent people into clients at all costs.

Unless it disabuses the client of his urge to demand and take more services, consumer protection only reinforces the collusion between giver and taker, and can play only a tactical and a transitory role in

---

[51]Tom Dewar, "Some Notes on the Professionalization of the Client," CIDOC Document I/V 73/37, Cuernavaca, 1973.

[52]Robert J. Haggerty, "The Boundaries of Health Care," *Pharos*, July 1972, pp. 106–11.

any political movement aimed at the health-oriented limitation of medicine. Consumer-protection movements can translate information about medical ineffectiveness now buried in medical journals into the language of politics, but they can make substantive contributions only if they develop into defense leagues for civil liberties and move beyond the control of quality and cost into the defense of untutored freedom to take or leave the goods. Any kind of dependence soon turns into an obstacle to autonomous mutual care, coping, adapting, and healing, and what is worse, into a device by which people are stopped from transforming the conditions at work and at home that make them sick. Control over the production side of the medical complex can work towards better health only if it leads to at least a very sizable reduction of its total output, rather than simply to technical improvements in the wares that are offered.

Equal Access to Torts

The most common and obvious political issue related to health is based on the charge that access to medical care is inequitable, that it favors the rich over the poor,[53] the influential over the powerless. While the level of medical services rendered to the members

---

[53]Health Policy Advisory Committee, *The American Health Empire: Power, Profits, and Politics,* ed., Barbara and John Ehrenreich (New York: Random House, 1970). Since the late 1960s the Health Policy Advisory Center, 17 Murray St., New York 10007, has played an important role in exposing those technical and organizational disorders built into the U.S. medical system as a consequence of its capitalist exploitative character. The *Health-PAC Bulletin,* published at the same address, is a valuable record of the evolution of this critique. The Ehrenreichs are probably representative of their group's thinking at the time of publication. The integration of a health profession, health industries, and government health bureaucracies promotes in each of these bodies characteristics typical of any transnational corporation. These common characteristics amalgamate them into a "complex" geared to reinforce infantile, racist, and sexist responses in those it pampers with subtle or gross arbitrariness. The elimination of the profit motive and wide participation by healthy and sick in policy-making would render the system accountable, equitable, and more effective for health care.

of technical elites does not vary significantly from one country to another, say from Sweden and Czechoslovakia to Indonesia and Senegal, the value of the services rendered to the typical citizen in different countries varies by factors exceeding the proportion of one to one thousand.[54] In many poor countries, the few are socially predetermined to get much more than the majority, not so much because they are rich as because they are children of soldiers or bureaucrats or because they live close to the one large hospital. In rich countries members of different minorities are underprivileged, not because, in terms of money per capita, they necessarily get less than their share,[55] but because they get substantially less than they have been trained to need. The slum dweller cannot reach the doctor when he needs him, and what is worse, the old, if they are poor and locked in a "home," cannot get away from him. For these and similar reasons, political parties convert the desire for health into demands for equal access to medical facilities.[56]

---

[54]In Upper Volta in Central Africa, about $25 million is spent annually for all medical services, including drugs, consumed within the country. Twice this amount in government expenditure goes to transport a few of the sick to Paris and to hospitalize them there. This compares with a total grant-in-aid for all nonmilitary purposes of $50 million yearly by France to its ex-colony. From the ever impeccably informed humor sheet for French bureaucrats, *Le Canard enchainé*, January 1, 1975.

[55]Nathan Glazer, "Paradoxes of Health Care," *Public Interest* 22 (winter 1971): 62–77. Low-income families in the U.S. receive not less but more health dollars than the income group immediately above them.

[56]For a framework useful in the creation of needs, see Jonathan Bradshaw, "A Taxonomy of Social Need," in Gordon McLachlan, ed., *Problems and Progress in Medical Care: Essays on Current Research* (New York: Oxford University Press, 1972), 7:69–82. To clarify and make explicit what is done when bureaucrats concerned with a social service plan to meet a social need, Bradshaw distinguishes 12 distinct situations according to the presence or absence of any of four need-factors: (1) *normative need,* defined by expert or professional knowledge; (2) *felt need,* defined by want; (3) *expressed need,* or demand; (4) *comparative need,* obtained by studying the characteristics of a population in receipt of service (those with similar characteristics not in receipt of service are then defined as standing in need). See also Kenneth Boulding, "The Concept of Need for Health Services," *Milbank Memorial Fund Quarterly* 44

They usually do not question the goods the medical system produces but insist that their constituents have a right to all that is produced for the privileged.[57]

In the poor countries, the poor majorities clearly have less access to medical services than the rich:[58] the services available to the few consume most of the health budget and deprive the majority of services of any kind. In all of Latin America, except Cuba, only one child in forty from the poorest fifth of the population finishes the five years of compulsory schooling;[59] a similar proportion of the poor can expect hospital treatment if they become seriously ill. In Venezuela, one day in a hospital costs ten times the average daily income; in Bolivia, about forty times the average daily income.[60] Everywhere in Latin America, the rich constitute the 3 percent of the population who are college graduates, labor

---

(October 1966): 202–23. For Richard M. Titmuss's testament on this subject, see *Social Policy: An Introduction* (New York: Pantheon Books, 1975), especially chap. 10, "Values and Choices," pp. 132–41.

[57]Kadushin, "Social Class and the Experience of Ill Health." Members of the upper class are always more competent in making use of publicly financed medical services, because of their greater sophistication and sometimes because of their ability to use small payments for gaining leverage on large perquisites.

[58]Jesús M. de Miguel, "Framework for the Study of National Health Systems," paper submitted to the Eighth World Congress of Sociology, August 1974, mimeographed. Tries to link regional differences within nations to the analysis of differences across nations. See table 1 for a chronotypology of comparative health systems research since 1930. Kerr L. White et al., "International Comparisons of Medical-Care Utilization," *New England Journal of Medicine* 277 (1967): 516–22. White points to the methodological difficulties involved in simultaneous measurements of a dependent variable like "utilization" in settings as different as England, Yugoslavia, and the U.S.A.

[59]David Barkin, "Access to and Benefits from Higher Education in Mexico," preliminary draft for comments. CIDOC Document A/E. 285, Cuernavaca, 1970.

[60]Arnoldo Gabaldón, "Health Service and Socio-economic Development in Latin America," *Lancet*, 1969, 1:739–44. Gunnar Adler-Karlsson, "Unequal Access to Health Within and Between Nations," paper written for the Gottlieb Duttweiler Institute's Symposium on "The Limits to Medicine," Davos, March 24–26, 1975, mimeographed.

leaders, political party officials, and members of families who have access to services either through money or simply through connections. These few receive costly treatment, often from the doctors of their choice. Most of the physicians, who come from the same social class as their patients, were trained to international standards on government grants.[61]

Notwithstanding unequal access to hospital care, the availability of medical service does not inevitably correlate with personal income. In Mexico about 3 percent of the population has access to the Instituto de Seguridad y Servicios Sociales de las Trabajadores del Estado (ISSSTE), that special part of the social security system which still holds a record for combining personal nursing care with advanced technological sophistication. This fortunate group is made up of government employees who receive truly equal treatment, whether they are ministers or office boys, and can count on high-quality care because they are part of a demonstration model. The newspapers, accordingly, inform the schoolmaster in a remote village that Mexican surgery is as well endowed as its counterpart in Chicago and that the surgeons who operate on him measure up to the standards of their colleagues in Houston. When high-level officials are hospitalized, they may be annoyed because for the first time in their lives they have to share a hospital room with a workman, but they are also proud of the high level of socialist commitment their nation shows in providing the same for boss and custodian. Both kinds of patient tend to overlook the fact that they are equally privileged exploiters. Providing the 3 percent with beds, equipment, administration, and technical care takes one-third of the public-health-care budget of the entire country. To be able to afford to give all of the poor equal access to medicine of uniform quality in poor countries, most of the present training and

---

[61] Joseph ben David, "Professions in the Class System of Present-Day Societies: A Trend Report and Bibliography," *Current Sociology* 12 (1963–64): 247–330.

activity of the health professions would have to be discontinued. However, delivery of effective basic health services for the entire population is cheap enough to be bought for everyone, provided no one could get more, regardless of the social, economic, medical, or personal reasons advanced for special treatment. If priority were given to equity in poor countries and service limited to the basics of effective medicine, entire populations would be encouraged to share in the demedicalization of modern health care and to develop the skills and confidence for self-care, thus protecting their countries from social iatrogenic disease.

In the rich countries, the economics of health are somewhat different.[62] At first sight, concern for the poor appears to demand further increases in the total health budget.[63] Yet the more people come to depend on care by service institutions, the more difficult it is to identify equity with equal access and equal benefits.[64] Is equity realized when equal numbers of

---

[62]For a simplified visual representation, Elizah L. White, "A Graphic Presentation on Age and Income Differentials in Selected Aspects of Morbidity, Disability and Utilization of Health Services," *Inquiry* 5, no. 1 (1968): 18–30. For a more detailed and up-to-date analysis, R. Anderson and John F. Newman, "Societal and Individual Determinants of Health Care in the U.S.A." *Milbank Memorial Fund Quarterly* 51 (winter 1973): 95–124.

[63]On the link between poverty and ill-health in the U.S., see John Kosa et al., eds., *Poverty and Health: A Sociological Analysis,* a Commonwealth Fund Book (Cambridge, Mass.: Harvard Univ. Press, 1969). This collection of papers is a plea for federal health insurance. Herbert T. Birch and Joan Dye Gussow, *Disadvantaged Children: Health, Nutrition and School Failure* (New York: Harcourt Brace, 1970). Though the authors believe in the value of more medical care for the poor, the non-treatment-related factors that discriminate against the health of poor children are indicated as being by far the most important.

[64]The relationship of mortality to both medical care and environmental variables is examined in a regression analysis by Richard Auster et al., "The Production of Health: An Exploratory Study," *Journal of Human Resources* 4 (fall 1969): 411–36. If education and medical care are controlled, high income is associated with high morality. This probably reflects unfavorable diet, lack of exercise, and psychological tension in the richer groups. Adverse factors associated with the growth of income may nullify the beneficial effects

dollars are available for the education of rich and poor? Or does it require that the poor get the same "education" although more will have to be spent on their account to achieve equal results? Or must the educational system, in order to be equitable, assure that the poor are not humiliated and hurt more than the rich with whom they compete on the academic ladder? Or is equity in learning opportunities provided only when all citizens share the same kind of learning environment? This battle of equity versus equality in the access to institutional care, already being waged in education, is now shaping up in the medical field.[65] In contrast to education, however, the issue in health can easily be resolved on available evidence. The per capita expenditure on health care, even for the poorest sector within the United States population, indicates that the base line at which such care turns iatrogenic has long since been passed. In rich countries, the total budget of services for the poor, if used for that which reinforces self-care, is more than ample. More access, even though restricted to those who now receive less, would only equalize the delivery of professional illusions and torts.

There are two aspects to health: freedom and rights. Above all, health designates the range of autonomy within which a person exercises control over his own biological states and over the conditions of his immediate environment. In this sense, health is identical with the degree of lived freedom. Primarily the law ought to guarantee the equitable distribution of health as freedom, which, in turn, depends on environmental conditions that only organized political

---

of an increase in the quantity and quality of medical care. Special risks for the superrich are not something entirely new. S. Gilfillan, "Roman Culture and Systemic Lead Poisoning," *Mankind Quarterly* 5 (January 1965): 55–9. Analysis of bones from 3rd-century Roman cemeteries revealed high concentrations of lead. The poisoning was probably due to the lead used for sealing amphoras in which wine was imported from Greece.

[65]Rashi Fein, "On Achieving Access and Equity in Health Care," *Milbank Memorial Fund Quarterly* 50 (October 1972): 34.

efforts can achieve. Beyond a certain level of intensity, health care, however, equitably distributed, will smother health-as-freedom. In this fundamental sense, health care is a matter of well-ordered liberty. Implicit in this concept is a preferred position of inalienable freedoms to do certain things, and here civil liberty must be distinguished from civil rights. The liberty to act without restraint from government has a wider scope than the civil rights the state may enact to guarantee that people will have equal powers to obtain certain goods or services.

Civil liberties ordinarily do not force others to carry out my wishes; a person may publish his or her opinion freely as far as the government is concerned, but this does not imply a duty for any one newspaper to print that opinion. A person may need to drink wine in his kind of worship, but no mosque has to welcome him to do so within its walls. At the same time, the state as a guarantor of liberties can enact laws that protect equal rights without which its members would not enjoy their freedoms. Such rights give meaning to equality, while liberties give shape to freedom. One sure way to extinguish freedom to speak, to learn, or to heal is to delimit them by transmogrifying civil rights into civic duties. The freedoms of the self-taught will be abridged in an overeducated society just as the freedom to health care can be smothered by overmedicalization. Any sector of the economy can be so expanded that for the sake of more costly levels of equality, freedoms are extinguished.

We are concerned here with movements that try to remedy the effects of socially iatrogenic medicine through political and legal control of the management, allocation, and organization of medical activities. Insofar as medicine is a public utility, however, no reform can be effective unless it gives priority to two sets of limits. The first relates to the volume of institutional treatment any individual can claim: no person is to receive services so extensive that his treatment deprives others of an opportunity for considerably less costly care per capita if, in their judgment (and not just in the opinion of an expert), they make a request of comparable urgency for the same public resources. Conversely, no services are to be forcibly imposed on an individual against his will: no man, without his consent, shall be seized, imprisoned, hospitalized, treated, or otherwise molested in the name of health. The second set of limits relates to the medical enterprise as a whole. Here the idea of health-as-freedom has to restrict the total output of health services within subiatrogenic limits that maximize the synergy of autonomous and heteronomous modes of health production. In democratic societies, such limitations are probably unachievable without guarantees of equity—without equal access. In that sense, the politics of equity is probably an essential element of an effective program for health. Conversely, if concern with equity is not linked to constraints on total production, and if it is not used as a countervailing force to the expansion of institutional medical care, it will be futile.[66]

Public Controls over the Professional Mafia

A third category of political remedies for unhealthy medicine focuses directly on *how* doctors do their work. Like consumer advocacy and legislation of access, this attempt to impose lay control on the medical organization has inevitable health-denying effects when it is changed from an ad hoc tactic into a general strategy.,

Four and a half million men and women in two hundred occupations are employed in the production and delivery of medically approved health services in the United States. (Only 8 percent are physicians,

---

[66]Emanuel de Kadt, "Inequality and Health," Univ. of Sussex, January 1975, goes far beyond most other authors in stressing the point I want to make: "Professional ideologies that focus on the maintenance of high standards of medical care keep in being a health system which neglects the simple needs of the many in order to concentrate on the complex and costly conditions of a few" (pp. 5 and 24).

whose net income after deductions for rent, personnel, and supplies represents 15 percent of total health expenditures and whose average income in 1973 was $50,000.[67]) The total does not include osteopaths, chiropractors, and others who might have specialized university training and require a license to practice, but who, unlike pharmacists, optometrists, laboratory technicians, and similar physicians' underlings, do not produce health care of the same prestige.[68] Even further removed from the establishment, and therefore excluded from these statistics, are thousands of purveyors of nonconventional health care, ranging from mail-order herbalists and masseurs to teachers of yoga.[69]

Of the many claimants to competence who are more or less integrated into the official establishment, about thirty categories are licensed in the United States.[70] In no state of the union is a license required

---

[67]For the medical enterprise at the service of specialization, see Rosemary Stevens, *American Medicine and the Public Interest* (New Haven, Conn.: Yale Univ. Press, 1973). For the parallel in Germany: Hans-Heinz Eulner, "Die Entwicklung der medizinischen Spezialfächer an den Universitäten des deutschen Sprachgebietes," in *Studien zur Medizingeschichte des 19. Jh.* (Stuttgart: Enke, 1970).

[68]Howard Freeman, Sol Levine and Leo Reeder, *Handbook of Medical Sociology* (Englewood Cliffs, N.J.: Prentice-Hall, 1963), pp. 216–17, for information on the relative number of qualified chiropractors and physicians (1 to 10), on the first university-affiliated colleges for physicians (1765), dentists (1868), and optometrists (1901).

[69]Michael Marien, "The Psychic Frontier: Toward New Paradigms for Man: Guide to 200 Books, Articles, and Journals," draft, March 1974, World Institute Council, 777 United Nations Plaza, New York 10017. A reading guide to about 200 recent books, journals, and institute newsletters, many with indications of content and evaluations, all concerned with alternate modes of staying healthy or healing. Can give to the uninitiated to this area a sense of the spectrum from the doctrinaire to the serious and the pompous. Academy of Parapsychology and Medicine, *The Dimensions of Healing: A Symposium* (Los Altos, Calif.: the Academy, 1972). Sheila Ostrander and Lynn Schroeder, *Psychic Discoveries Behind the Iron Curtain* (Englewood Cliffs, N.J.: Prentice-Hall, 1970; New York: Bantam, 1971).

[70]Henry E. Sigerist, "The History of Medical Licensure," *Journal of the American Medical Association* 104 (1935): 1057–60, on the transition from occupational pluralism to the professional dominance

for fewer than fourteen kinds of practitioners.[71] These licenses are issued on completion of formal educational programs and sometimes on the evidence of a successful examination; in rare instances, proficiency or experience is a prerequisite for admission to independent practice.[72] Competent or successful work is nowhere a condition for continuing in practice. Renewal is automatic, usually upon payment of a fee; only fifteen out of fifty states permit a physician's license to be challenged on grounds of incompetence.[73] While claims to specialist standing come and go on the fringes, the specialties recognized by the American Medical Association have steadily increased, doubling in the last fifteen years: half the practicing American physicians are specialists in one of sixty categories, and the proportion is expected to increase to 55 percent before 1980.[74] Within each of these fields a fiefdom has developed with specialized nurses, technicians, journals, congresses, and sometimes organized groups of patients pressing for more public funds.[75] The cost of coordinating the treat-

---

of the new physician whose competence in "scientific" diagnosis and therapy was guaranteed by attendance at a medical school that had weathered Flexner's report.

[71]Ronald Akers and Richard Quinney, "Differential Organization of Health Professions: A Comparative Analysis," *American Sociological Review* 33 (February 1968): 104–21. On the internal social organization of licensed physicians, dentists, optometrists, pharmacists, and their relative cohesion, wealth, and power.

[72]William L. Frederick, "The History and Philosophy of Occupational Licensing Legislation in the United States," *Journal of the American Dental Association* 58 (March 1959): 18–25.

[73]U.S. Department of Health, Education, and Welfare, *Medical Malpractice*, Report of the Secretary's Commission on Medical Practice, January 16, 1973.

[74]Health Services Research Center, Institute for Interdisciplinary Studies, Medical Manpower Specialty Distribution Project 1975–80, working paper 1971.

[75]For studies on the limits to further proliferation, see William J. Goode, "The Theoretical Limits of Professionalization," in Amitai Etzioni, ed., *The Semi-Professions and Their Organization* (New York: Free Press, 1969), pp. 266–313. Goode believes that though techniques continue to multiply, fewer of them require for their

ment of the same patient by several specialists grows exponentially with each added competence, as does the risk of mistakes and the probability of damage due to the unexpected combination of different therapies. As the number of patient relationships outgrows the elements in the total population, the occupations dealing with medical information, insurance, and patient defense multiply unchecked. Of course, physicians lord it over these fiefs and determine what work these pseudo-professions shall do. But with the recognition of some autonomy many of these specialized groups of medical pages, ushers, footmen, and squires have also gained some power to evaluate how well they do their own work. By gaining the right to self-evaluation according to special criteria that fit its own view of reality, each new specialty generates for society at large a new impediment to evaluating what its work actually contributes to the health of patients. Organized medicine has practically ceased to be the art of healing the curable, and consoling the hopeless has turned into a grotesque priesthood concerned with salvation and has become a law unto itself. The policies that promise the public some control over the medical endeavor tend to overlook the fact that to achieve their purpose they must control a church, not an industry.

Dozens of concrete strategies are now being discussed and proposed to make the health industry more health-serving and less-self-serving: decentralization of delivery; universal public insurance; group practice by specialists; health-maintenance programs

---

execution that trust on the part of the client on which professional autonomy is built. Further specialization of competence might therefore concentrate professional power again in fewer hands. See also Wilbert Moore and Gerald W. Rosenblum, *The Professions: Roles and Rules* (New York: Russell Sage, 1970), chap. 3. Harold Wilensky, "The Professionalization of Everyone?" *American Journal of Sociology* 70 (September 1964): 137–58. The process of professionalization cannot be extrapolated, because bureaucratization threatens the ideal of dedicated service even more intensely than it undermines the autonomy of the one who performs services.

rather than sick-care; payment of a fixed amount per patient per year (capitation) rather than fee-for-service; elimination of present restrictions on the use of health manpower; more rational organization and utilization of the hospital system; replacement of the licensing of individuals by the licensing of institutions held to performance standards; and the organization of patient cooperatives to balance or support a professional medical power.

Each of these proposals would indeed improve medical efficiency, but at the cost of a further decline in society's effective health care. To increase efficiency by upward mobility of personnel and downward assignment of responsibility could not but tighten the integration of the medical-care industry and with it social polarization.

As the training of middle-level professionals becomes more expensive, nursing personnel in the lower ranks is becoming scarce. Poor salaries, growing disdain for servant and housekeeping roles, an increase in chronic patients (and consequent growing tedium in their care), disappearance of the religious motivation for nuns and deacons, and new opportunities for women in other fields all contribute to a manpower crisis. In England nearly two-thirds of all low-level hospital personnel come from overseas, usually from former colonies; in Germany, from Turkey and Yugoslavia; in France, from North Africa; in the United States, from racial minorities. The creation of new ranks, titles, curricula, roles, and specialties at the bottom level is a doubtfully effective remedy. The hospital only reflects the labor economy of a high-technology society: transnational specialization on the top, bureaucracies in the middle, and at the bottom, a a new subproletariat made up of migrants and the professionalized client.[76]

The multiplication of paraprofessional specialists

---

[76]For the current crisis in the U.S. nursing profession, see National Commission for the Study of Nursing Education, *An Abstract for Action* (New York: McGraw-Hill, 1970).

further decreases what the diagnostician does for the person who seeks his help, while the multiplication of generalist auxiliaries tends to reduce what uncertified people may do for each other or for themselves.[77] Institutional licensing[78] would indeed permit a more efficient deployment of personnel, a more rational health-manpower mix, and greater opportunity for advancement: it would no doubt greatly improve the delivery of medical staples such as dental work, bonesetting, and the delivery of babies. But if it became the model for over-all health care, it would be equivalent to the creation of a medical Ma Bell.[79] Lay control over an expanding medical technocracy is not unlike the professionalization of the patient: both enhance medical power and increase its *nocebo* effect. As long as the public bows to the professional monopoly in assigning the sick-role, it cannot control hidden health hierarchies that multiply patients.[80]

---

[77]The autonomous and independent health technician, free of control by the medical hierarchy, is still taboo: Oscar Gish, ed., *Health, Manpower and the Medical Auxiliary: Some Notes and an Annotated Bibliography*, Intermediate Technology Development Group (London, 1971). Gish tries to distinguish between the costly, prestigious, intensely skilled professional, with his long training and his readiness to move away from the community; the paraprofessional nurse, whose training is academic and theoretical; and the health auxiliary, who has the skills that are needed most of the time.

[78]Victor Fuchs, *Who Shall Live? Health Economics and Social Choice* (New York: Basic Books, 1974). Nathan Hershey and Walter S. Wheeler, *Health Personnel Regulation in the Public Interest: Questions and Answers on Institutional Licensure*, published by the California Hospital Association as a service to the health-care field, 1973.

[79]S. Kelman, "Towards a Political Economy of Medical Care," *Inquiry* 8, no. 3 (1971): 30–8. Kelman claims that the predominance of financial capital in the health sector might foreshadow a decline in the autonomy of the professional, as he is forced to unionize. Institutional licensing, which would turn even the medical-team captain into an employee, would certainly accentuate this trend. Compare this with note 75, p. 242 above.

[80]Corinne Lathrop Gilb, *Hidden Hierarchies: The Professions and Government* (New York: Harper & Row, 1966). On the strategies used by American physicians, lawyers, and educators to acquire political power by organizing professional associations and by claiming as a right what, at the outset, had been an honored prerogative.

The medical clergy can be controlled only if the law is used to restrict and disestablish its monopoly on deciding what constitutes disease, who is sick, and what ought to be done to him or her.[81]

Misdirection of blame for iatrogenesis is the most serious political obstacle to public control over health care. To turn doctor-baiting into radical chic would be the surest way to defuse any political crisis fueled by the new health consciousness. If physicians were to become conspicuous scapegoats, the gullible patient would be relieved from blame for his therapeutic greed. School-baiting did save the institutional enterprise when crisis last hit in education. The same strategy could now save the medical system and keep it essentially as it is.

Quite suddenly in the 1970s the schools lost their status as sacred cows. Driven by Sputnik, racial conflict, and new frontiers, the school bubble had outgrown all nonmilitary budgets and had burst. For a short while, the hidden curriculum of the school system lay exposed. It became conventional wisdom that after a certain point in its expansion, the school system inevitably reproduces a meritocratic class society and neatly arranges people according to levels of highly specialized torpor for which they are trained in graded, age-specific, competitive, and compulsory rituals. Frustration of an expensive dream had led many people to grasp that no amount of compulsory learning could equitably prepare the young for industrial hierarchies, and that all effective preparation of children for an inhuman socio-economic system constituted systematic aggression against their persons. At this point a new vision of reality could have grown into a radical revolt against a capital-intensive

---

[81]I owe the idea that professions are based on a grant to Eliot Freidson, *Profession of Medicine: A Study of the Sociology of Applied Knowledge* (New York: Dodd, Mead, 1971), whom I follow closely. For an orientation on the status of the discussion, besides Freidson see Howard S. Becker, "The Nature of Profession," in Henry Nelson, ed., *Education for the Professions* (Chicago: National Society for the Study of Education, 1962), chap. 2, pp. 27–46.

system of production and the beliefs that bolster it. But instead of blaming the hubris of pedagogues, the public conceded to pedagogues more power to do precisely as they pleased. Disgruntled teachers focused criticism on their peers, the methods, the organization of schooling, and the financing of institutions, all of which were defined as obstacles to effective education.

School-baiting enabled liberal schoolmasters to mutate into a new breed of adult educators. School-baiting not only saved but—momentarily—upgraded the salary and prestige of the teacher. Whereas before the crisis point the schoolmaster had been restricted in his pedagogical aggression to an age-specific group below sixteen years of age, which was exposed to him during class hours in the school building to be initiated into a limited number of subjects, the new knowledge-merchant now considers the world his classroom. While the curricular teacher could disqualify only those nonstudents who dared to learn a curricular matter on their own, the new manager of lifelong and recurrent "education," "conscientization," "sensitivity training," or "politicization" presumes to degrade in the eyes of the public any behavioral patterns that he has not approved. The school-baiting of the sixties could easily set the pattern for the coming medical war. Following the lead of the teachers who declare that the world is their classroom, some chic crusading physicians[82] now jump onto the bandwagon of medicine-baiting and channel public frustration and anger at curative medicine into a call for a new elite of scien-

---

[82]Howard S. Becker, *Outsiders: Studies in the Sociology of Deviance* (New York: Free Press, 1963), p. 177, points out that the most obvious consequence of a successful crusade against some evil is the creation of a set of new rules and established officials to enforce them. "Just as radical political movements turn into organized political parties and lusty evangelical sects become staid religious denominations," so, I argue here, people who have started out to materialize dreams of health delivery turn into a profession of wardens.

tific guardians who would control the world as their ward.[83]

The Scientific Organization—of Life

Belief in medicine as an applied science generates a fourth kind of countermeasure to iatrogenesis which inevitably increases the irresponsible power of the health profession—and thereby the damage medicine does. The proponents of higher scientific standards in medical research and social organization argue that pathogenic medicine is due to the overwhelming number of bad doctors let loose on society. Fewer decision-makers, more carefully screened, better trained, more tightly supervised by their peers, and more effectively in command over what is done for whom and how, would ensure that the powerful resources now available to medical scientists would be

---

[83]Vicente Navarro, "Social Policy Issues: An Explanation of the Composition, Nature, and Functions of the Present Health Sector of the United States," Johns Hopkins University, paper based on a presentation at the Annual Conference of the New York Academy of Medicine, April 25–26, 1974. Navarro argues that the prevailing values in the health sector are indeed shaped by the health establishment, but are symptomatic of the distribution of economic and political power within society. The power to shape health values gives the professionals within the health sector a dominant influence on the structure of the health services, but actually no control. This control is exercised through the ownership of the means of production, reproduction, and legitimation held by the capitalist elite. Navarro does not seem to realize that I do agree with him on this point but am less naïvely optimistic as to the political indifference of each and every *technique* used in the provision of health care. I argue that dialysis, transplants, and intensive care for most chronic diseases, but also just the general intensity of our medical endeavor, inevitably impose exploitation on any society that wants to use them in the repertory of its medical-care system. See Vicente Navarro, "The Industrialization of Fetishism or the Fetishism of Industrialization: A Critique of Ivan Illich," Johns Hopkins University, January 1975. For the argument that medical ideologies shape a care system that they do not control, see also Massimo Gaglio, *Medicina e profitto: Tesi di discussione per operai, studenti e tecnici* (Milan: Sapere Editore, 1971), and Aloisi et al., *La medicina e la societá contemporanea,* Atti del Convegno promoso dall'Instituto Gramsci, Roma, 28–30 giugno 1967. (Rome: Editori Riuniti, 1968).

applied for the benefit of the people.[84] Such idolatry of science overlooks the fact that research conducted as if medicine were an ordinary science, diagnosis conducted as if patients were specific cases and not autonomous persons, and therapy conducted by hygienic engineers are the three approaches which coalesce into the present endemic health-denial.

As a science, medicine lies on a borderline. Scientific method provides for experiments conducted on models. Medicine, however, experiments not on models but on the subjects themselves. But medicine tells us as much about the meaningful performance of healing, suffering, and dying as chemical analysis tells us about the aesthetic value of pottery.[85]

In the pursuit of applied science the medical profession has largely ceased to strive towards the goals of an association of artisans who use tradition, experience, learning and intuition, and has come to play a role reserved to ministers of religion, using scientific principles as its theology and technologists as acolytes.[86] As an enterprise, medicine is now concerned less with the empirical art of healing the curable and much more with the rational approach to the salvation of mankind from attack by illness, from the shackles of impairment, and even from the neces-

---

[84]Philip Selby, "Health in 1980–1990: A Predictive Study Based on an International Inquiry," *Perspectives in Medicine,* vol. 6 (1974). Forecast, based on a Delphi scenario, describing a utopia that fits the desires of the six dozen health bureaucrats interviewed.

[85]Owing to this fact, the innocence of scientific research is absent from medicine. Hans Jonas, "Philosophical Reflections on Experimenting with Human Subjects," in Paul A. Freund, ed., *Experimentation with Human Subjects* (New York: Braziller, 1969), pp. 1–28. Although this article deals primarily with extreme forms of experimentation, it provides a lucid introduction to the relationship between experiment and service.

[86]Harris L. Coulter, *Divided Legacy. A History of the Schism in Medical Thought,* vol. 1, *The Patterns Emerge: Hippocrates to Paracelsus;* vol. 2, *Progress and Regress: J. B. Van Helmont to Claude Bernard;* vol. 3, *Science and Ethics in American Medicine: 1800–1914* (Washington, D.C.: McGrath, 1973). A vast and well-documented recent attempt to paint the history of empirical medicine in constant tension with the rationalist tradition.

sity of death.[87] By turning from art to science, the body of physicians has lost the traits of a guild of craftsmen applying rules established to guide the masters of a practical art for the benefit of actual sick persons. It has become an orthodox apparatus of bureaucratic administrators who apply scientific principles and methods to whole categories of medical cases. In other words, the clinic has turned into a laboratory. By claiming predictable outcomes without considering the human performance of the healing person and his integration in his own social group, the modern physician has assumed the traditional posture of the quack.

As a member of the medical profession the individual physician is an inextricable part of a scientific team. Experiment is the method of science, and the records he keeps—if he likes it or not—are part of the data for a scientific enterprise. Each treatment is one more repetition of an experiment with a statistically known probability of success. As in any operation that constitutes a genuine application of science, failure is said to be due to some sort of ignorance: insufficient knowledge of the laws that apply in the particular experimental situation, a lack of personal competence in the application of method and principles on the part of the experimenter, or else his inability to control that elusive variable which is the patient himself. Obviously, the better the patient can be controlled, the more predictable will be the outcome in this kind of medical endeavor. And the more predictable the outcome on a population basis, the more effective will the organization appear to be. The technocrats of medicine tend to promote the interests of science rather than the needs of society.[88] The

---

[87] Henry E. Sigerist, "Probleme der medizinischen Historiographie," *Sudhoffs Archiv* 24 (1931); 1–18. The history of medicine can be written as a history of disease patterns, medical ideologies, or medical activities. The first two approaches are often neglected.

[88] The argument is strongly formulated by Gerald Leach, *The Biocrats: Implications of Medical Progress* (New York: McGraw-Hill, 1970; rev. ed., Baltimore: Penguin, 1972).

practitioners corporately constitute a research bureaucracy. Their primary responsibility is to science in the abstract or, in a nebulous way, to their profession.[89] Their personal responsibility for the particular client has been resorbed into a vague sense of power extending over all tasks and clients of all colleagues. Medical science applied by medical scientists provides the correct treatment, regardless of whether it results in a cure, or death sets in, or there is no reaction on the part of the patient. It is legitimized by statistical tables, which predict all three outcomes with a certain frequency. The individual physician in a concrete case may still remember that he owes nature and the patient as much gratitude as the patient owes him if he has been successful in the use of his art. But only a high level of tolerance for cognitive dissonance will allow him to carry on in the divergent roles of healer and scientist.[90]

The proposals that seek to counter iatrogenesis by eliminating the last vestiges of empiricism from the encounter between the patient and the medical system are latter-day crusaders of an inquisitorial

---

[89]Talcott Parsons, "Research with Human Subjects and the 'Professional complex,'" in Freund, *Experimentation with Human Subjects,* pp. 116 ff. Parsons distinguishes within the medical-professional complex (1) research, concerned with the creation of new knowledge; (2) service, which utilizes knowledge for practical human interests; and (3) teaching, which transmits knowledge. He argues that the laity needs formal recognition of the right to minimize injuries resulting from unresolved tensions in this complex.

[90]After the patient has been damaged or has died, the physician will try to freeze the decision that led to this result by reducing *cognitive dissonance.* The argument in favor of the alternative he has chosen appears ever stronger as he represses the arguments in favor of the unchosen alternative. He is acting like a housewife: before she goes out to shop, the more expensive the food, the less likely it is to get to the family table; after her visit to the supermarket and her decision to buy, the higher the cost, the more likely the food is to be used. See Leon Festinger, *Conflict, Decision, and Dissonance,* Stanford Studies in Psychology no. 3 (Stanford, Calif.: Stanford Univ. Press, 1964). On the role conflict between the physician as adviser and the physician as scientist see Eliot Freidson, *Professional Dominance: The Social Structure of Medical Care* (Chicago: Aldine, 1972).

kind.[91] They use the religion of scientism to devalue political judgment. While operational verification in the laboratory is the measure of science, the contest of adversaries appealing to a jury that applies past experience to a present issue, as this issue is experienced by actual persons, constitutes the measure of politics. By denying public recognition to entities that cannot be measured by science, the call for pure, orthodox, confirmed medical practice shields this practice from all political evaluation.

The religious preference given to scientific language over the language of the layman is one of the major bulwarks of professional privilege. The imposition of this specialized language upon political discourse about medicine easily voids it of effectiveness.

The deprofessionalization of medicine does not imply the proscription of technical language any more than it calls for the exclusion of genuine competence, nor does it oppose public scrutiny and exposure of malpractice. But it does imply a bias against the mystification of the public, against the mutual accreditation of self-appointed healers, against the public support of a medical guild and of its institutions, and against the legal discrimination by, and on behalf of, people whom individuals or communities choose and appoint as their healers. The deprofessionalization of medicine does not mean denial of public funds for curative purposes, but it does mean a bias against the disbursement of any such funds under the prescription or control of guild members. It does not mean the abolition of modern medicine. It means

---

[91] Allan Hoffman and David Rittenhouse Inglis, "Radiation and Infants," review of *Low-Level Radiation*, by Ernest J. Sternglass, *Bulletin of the Atomic Scientists*, December 1972, pp. 45–52. The reviewers foresee an imminent antiscientific backlash from the general public when the evidence provided by Sternglass becomes generally known. The public will come to feel it has been lulled into a sense of security by the unfounded optimism of the spokesmen for scientific institutions regarding the threat constituted by low-level radiation. The reviewers argue for policy research to prevent such a backlash and to protect the scientific community from its consequences.

that no professional shall have the power to lavish on any one of his patients a package of curative resources larger than that which any other could claim for his own. Finally, it does not mean disregard for the special needs that people manifest at special moments in their lives: when they are born, break a leg, become crippled, or face death. The proposal that doctors not be licensed by an in-group does not mean that their services shall not be evaluated, but rather that this evaluation can be done more effectively by informed clients than by their own peers. Refusal of direct funding to the more costly technical devices of medical magic does not mean that the state shall not protect individual people against exploitation by ministers of medical cults; it means only that tax funds shall not be used to establish any such rituals. Deprofessionalization of medicine means the unmasking of the myth according to which technical progress demands the solution of human problems by the application of scientific principles, the myth of benefit through an increase in the specialization of labor, through multiplication of arcane manipulations, and the myth that increasing dependence of people on the right of access to impersonal institutions is better than trust in one another.

Engineering for a Plastic Womb

So far I have dealt with four categories of criticism directed at the institutional structure of the medical-industrial complex. Each gives rise to a specific kind of political demand, and all of them become reinforcements for the dependence of people on medical bureaucracies because they deal with health care as a form of therapeutic planning and engineering.[92]

---

[92]Thomas M. Dunaye, "Health Planning: A Bibliography of Basic Readings," Council of Planning Librarians, Exchange Bibliography, mimeographed (Monticello, Ill., 1968), says: "So extensive is the literature of source materials on the subject of health planning that to provide a complete bibliography has become an elephantine problem. This difficulty has been partially overcome by the assembly

They indicate strategies for surgical, chemical, and behavioral intervention in the lives of sick people or people threatened with sickness. A fifth category of criticism rejects these objectives. Without relinquishing the view of medicine as an engineering endeavor, these critics assert that medical strategies fail because they concentrate too much effort on sickness and too little on changing the environment that makes people sick.

Most research on alternatives to clinical intervention is directed towards program engineering for the professional systems of man's social, psychological, and physical environment. "Non-health-service health determinants" are largely concerned with planned intervention in the milieu.[93] Therapeutic engineers

---

of separate bibliographies . . . many of which are included [in this] unified body of basic readings useful to the . . . newcomer to the field." See also National Library of Medicine. *Selected References on Environmental Quality as It Relates to Health Since 1971*, National Library of Medicine, 8600 Rockville Pike, Bethesda, Md.; National Institute of Environmental Health Science, Triangle Park, London, *Environmental Health*, periodical since 1971; National Library of Medicine, *Environmental Biology and Medicine*, periodical since 1971; *Current Bibliography of Epidemiology*, American Public Health Association, 1740 Broadway, N.Y. 10019.

[93]As an example of this approach, see Monroe Lerner et al., "The Non-Health Services' Determinants of Health Levels: Conceptualization and Public Policy Implications," report of a subcommittee under the Carnegie Grant to the Medical Sociology Section, American Sociological Association, August 29, 1973, mimeographed. This draft provides a rationale for the extension of the health bureaucracies' mandate to all those matters which traditionally lie beyond its competence by arguing that they lie within its inherent powers. Faced with the need to identify the limits of its field, the committee decided: (1) it will deal with factors affecting health levels, or perceived as doing so, not with concepts, measurements of health levels, or externalities of health for improvement of sociocultural levels; (2) it will deal selectively with factors that affect populations at risk; (3) it will deal with prevention, maintenance and adaptation relating to chronic illness and disability, but only so long as these are not perceived as "health services"; (4) it will deal with the unintended ill-health caused by contact with the system for the delivery of personal health. See also *The Sources of Health: An Annotated Bibliography of Current Research Regarding the Nontherapeutic Determinants of Health,* Center for Urban Affairs, Northwestern University (Evanston, Ill., 1973).

shift the thrust of their interventions from the potential or actual patient towards the larger system of which he is imagined to be a part. Instead of manipulating the sick, they redesign the environment to ensure a healthier population.[94]

Health care as environmental hygenic engineering works within categories different from those of the clinical scientist. Its focus is survival rather than health in its opposition to disease; the impact of stress on populations and individuals rather than the performance of specific persons; the relationship of a niche in the cosmos to the human species with which it has evolved rather than the relationship between the aims of actual people and their ability to achieve them.[95]

---

[94]Hugh Iltis, Orie Loucks, and Peter Andrews, "Criteria for an Optimum Human Environment," *Bulletin of the Atomic Scientists,* January 1970, pp. 2–6. George L. Engel, "A Unified Concept of Health and Disease," *Perspectives in Biology and Medicine* 3 (summer 1960): 459–85.

[95]For a theoretical analysis of the health levels specified in these terms, see Aaron Antonovsky, "Breakdown: A Needed Fourth Step in the Conceptual Armamentarium of Modern Medicine," *Social Science and Medicine* 6 (October 1972): 537–44. He calls for a fourth category in the conceptual tools of modern medicine: the recognition of breakdown. So far medicine has developed three major concepts for the control of disease. First it was discovered that disease could be prevented by environmental public health measures, especially by exerting control over supplies of food and water. The second breakthrough came with the concept of immunization, preparing the individual for resistance. Both these approaches are based on the image of the dangerous agent. A third breakthrough came with the recognition of multiple causation: one succumbs to a given disease when a given agent interacts with a given host in a given environment; the task of medicine is to recognize and control these givens. According to Antonovsky, even Dubos does not go explicitly beyond this concept of multiple causation, even though he stresses the need to enhance man's capacity to adapt to the stress threatening in specific diseases. Antonovsky suggests the ulterior concept of breakdown, and a definition that permits this global concept to be made operational. For this purpose he proposes specifications for four factors common to all disease: (1) pain may be absent, mild, moderate, or severe; (2) handicap may be absent, distracting, moderate, or severe; (3) acute or chronic character can be assessed in six ways: no acute or chronic condition, mild-chronic but not degenerative, acute but not life-threatening, serious-chronic but not degenerative, serious-chronic-degenera-

In general, people are more the product of their environment than of their genetic endowment. This environment is being rapidly distorted by industrialization. Although man has so far shown an extraordinary capacity for adaptation, he has survived with very high levels of sublethal breakdown. Dubos[96] fears that mankind will be able to adapt to the stresses of the second industrial revolution and overpopulation just as it survived famines, plagues, and wars in the past. He speaks of this kind of survival with fear because adaptability, which is an asset for survival, is also a heavy handicap: the most common causes of disease are exacting adaptive demands. The health-care system, without any concern for the feelings of people and for their health, simply concentrates on the engineering of systems that minimize breakdowns.

Two foreseeable and sinister consequences of a shift from patient-oriented to milieu-oriented medicine are the loss of the sense of boundaries between distinct categories of deviance, and a new legitimacy for total treatment.[97] Medical care, industrial safety,

---

tive, or acute and life-threatening; and finally (4) disease can be recognized by the medical profession as requiring no help, watching, or therapy. Thus 288 possible breakdown types have been established. For the author, "a radically new question arises: what is the aetiology of breakdown? Is there some new constellation of factors which is a powerful predictor of breakdown?"

[96]René Dubos, *Man and His Environment: Biomedical Knowledge and Social Action*, Pan-American Health Organization Scientific Publication no. 131 (Washington, D.C., 1966). Alexander Mitscherlich, "Psychosomatische Anpassungsgefährdungen," in *Das beschädigte Leben: Diagnose und Therapie in einer Welt unabsehbarer Veränderungen; Ein Symposium geleitet und herausgegeben von Alexander Mitscherlich* (Munich: Piper, 1969), pp. 35–46. At which point does the physician turn into the unethical accomplice of a destructive environment? S. V. Boyden, ed., *Cultural Adaptation to Biological Maladjustment: The Impact of Civilization on the Biology of Man* (Canberra: Australian National Univ. Press, 1970).

[97]For reference see Robert Harris, *Health and Crime Abstracts 1960–1971*, Houston Project for the Early Prevention of Individual Violence (Houston: Univ. of Texas School of Public Health, 1972). William Morrow et al., *Behavior Therapy Bibliography 1951–1969, Annotated and Indexed*, University of Missouri Studies no. 54 Columbia: Univ. of Missouri Press, 1971).

health education, and psychic reconditioning are all different names for the human engineering needed to fit populations into engineering systems. As the health-delivery system continually fails to meet the demands made upon it, conditions now classified as illness may soon develop into aspects of criminal deviance and asocial behavior. The behavioral therapy used on convicts in the United States[98] and the Soviet Union's incarceration of political adversaries in mental hospitals[99] indicate the direction in which the integration of therapeutic professions might lead: an increased blurring of boundaries between therapies administered with a medical, educational, or ideological rationale.[100]

The time has come not only for public assessment of medicine but also for public disenchantment with those monsters generated by the dream of environmental engineering. If contemporary medicine aims at making it unnecessary for people to feel or to heal, eco-medicine promises to meet their alienated desire for a plastic womb.

---

[98]David J. Rothman et al., "An Historical Overview: Behavior Modification in Total Institutions," *Hastings Center Report* 5 (February 1975): 17–24. Roy G. Spece, Jr., "Conditioning and Other Technologies Used to 'Treat?', 'Rehabilitate?', 'Demolish?' Prisoners and Mental Patients," *Southern California Law Review* 45, no. 2 (1972): 616–84. A survey of the legal status in the U.S. of therapies that aim at the alteration of behavior.

[99]For a particularly sensitive autobiographical report circulated in the Samizdat and published in the original in *Grani,* no. 79, 1971, see G. M. Shimanoff, "Souvenirs de la Maison Rouge," *Esprit* 9 (September 1972): 320–62.

[100]D. A. Begelman, "The Ethics of Behavioral Control and a New Mythology," *Psychotherapy* 8, no. 2 (1971): 165–9.

8

The Recovery of Health

Much suffering has been man-made. The history of man is one long catalogue of enslavement and exploitation, usually told in the epics of conquerors or sung in the elegies of their victims. War is at the heart of this tale, war and the pillage, famine, and pestilence that came in its wake. But it was not until modern times that the unwanted physical, social, and psychological side-effects of so-called peaceful enterprises began to compete with war in destructive power.

Man is the only animal whose evolution has been conditioned by adaptation on more than one front. If he did not succumb to predators and forces of nature, he had to cope with use and abuse by others of his own kind. In his struggle with the elements and with his neighbor, his character and culture were formed, his instincts withered, and his territory was turned into a *home*.

Animals adapt through evolution in response to changes in their natural environment. Only in man does challenge become conscious and the response to difficult and threatening situations take the form of rational action and of conscious habit. Man can design his relations to nature and neighbor, and he is able to survive even when his enterprise has partly failed. He is the animal that can endure trials with patience and learn by understanding them. He is the sole being who can and must resign himself to limits when he becomes aware of them. A conscious response to painful sensations, to impairment, and to eventual death is part of man's coping ability. The capacity for revolt and for perseverance, for stubborn resistance and for resignation, are integral parts of human life and health.

But nature and neighbor are only two of the three frontiers on which man must cope. A third front where doom can threaten has always been recognized. To remain viable, man must also survive the dreams which so far myth has both shaped and controlled. Now society must develop programs to cope with the irrational desires of its most gifted members. To date, myth has fulfilled the function of setting limits to the materialization of greedy, envious, murderous dreams. Myth assured the common man of his safety on this third frontier if he kept within its bounds. Myth guaranteed disaster to those few who tried to outwit the gods. The common man perished from infirmity or from violence; only the rebel against the human condition fell prey to Nemesis, the envy of the gods.

Industrialized Nemesis

Prometheus was hero, not Everyman. Driven by radical greed (*pleonexia*), he trespassed beyond the limits of man (*aitia* and *mesotes*) and in unbounded presumption (*hubris*) stole fire from heaven.[1] He

---

[1]On the political use of divine envy, see Svend Ranulf, *The Jealousy of the Gods and Criminal Law in Athens,* trans. Annie J. Fausböll, 2 vols. (Copenhagen: Levin & Munksgaard, 1933–34). On hubris calling forth nemesis, see David Grene, *Greek Political Theory: The Image of Man in Thucydides and Plato* (Chicago: Univ. of Chicago Press, Phoenix Books, 1965; orig. *Man in His Pride*); and E. R. Dodds, *The Greeks and the Irrational* (Berkeley: Univ. of California Press, 1951), especially chap. 2. Irving Kenneth

thus inevitably brought Nemesis on himself. He was put into irons and chained to a Caucasian rock. An eagle preyed all day on his liver, and heartlessly healing gods kept him alive by regrafting his liver each night. Nemesis inflicted on him a kind of pain meant for demigods, not for men. His hopeless and unending suffering turned the hero into an immortal reminder of inescapable cosmic retaliation.

The social nature of nemesis has now changed. With the industrialization of desire and the engineering of corresponding ritual responses, hubris has spread. Unbounded material progress has become Everyman's goal. Industrial hubris has destroyed the mythical framework of limits to irrational fantasies, has made technical answers to mad dreams seem rational, and has turned the pursuit of destructive values into a conspiracy between purveyor and client. Nemesis for the masses is now the inescapable backlash of industrial progress. Modern nemeis is the material monster born from the overarching industrial dream. It has spread as far and as wide as universal schooling, mass transportation, industrial wage labor, and the medicalization of health.

Inherited myths have ceased to provide limits for action. If the species is to survive the loss of its traditional myths, it must learn to cope rationally and politically with its envious, greedy, and lazy dreams. Myth alone can do the job no more. Politically established limits to industrial growth will have to take the place of mythological boundaries. Political exploration and recognition of the necessary material conditions for survival, equity, and effectiveness will have to set limits to the industrial mode of production.

Nemesis has become structural and endemic. Increasingly, man-made misery is the by-product of enterprises that were supposed to protect ordinary

---

Zola. "In the Name of Health and Illness;" on some political consequences of medical influence. in: Social Science and Medicine, Feb. 1975, vol. 9 pp. 83–87 . . . the medical area is the arena of the example par excellence of today's identity crisis, the area where the *banality of evil* is best masked as a technical, scientific, objective process engineered for our own good.

people in their struggle with the inclemency of the environment and against the wanton injustice inflicted on them by the elite. The main source of pain, of disability, and of death is now engineered, albeit nonintentional, harassment. Our prevailing ailments, helplessness, and injustice are largely the side-effects of strategies for more and better education, better housing, a better diet, and better health.

A society that values planned teaching above autonomous learning cannot but teach man to keep his engineered place. A society that relies for locomotion on managed transport must do the same. Beyond a certain level, energy used for transportation immobilizes and enslaves the majority of nameless passengers and provides advantages only for the elite. No new fuel, technology, or public controls can keep the rising mobilization and acceleration of society from producing rising harriedness, programmed paralysis, and inequality. The same is true for agriculture. Beyond a certain level of capital investment in the growing and processing of food, malnutrition will become pervasive. The results of the Green Revolution will then rack the livers of consumers more thoroughly than Zeus's eagle. No biological engineering can prevent undernourishment and food poisoning beyond this point. What is happening in the sub-Saharan Sahel is only a dress rehearsal for encroaching world famine. This is but the application of a general law: When more than a certain proportion of value is produced by the industrial mode, subsistence activities are paralyzed, equity declines, and total satisfaction diminishes. It will not be the sporadic famine that formerly came with drought and war, or the occasional food shortage that could be remedied by good will and emergency shipments. The coming hunger is a by-product of the inevitable concentration of industrialized agriculture in rich countries and in the fertile regions of poor countries. Paradoxically, the attempt to counter famine by further increases in industrially efficient agriculture only widens the scope of the catastrophe by depressing the use of marginal lands. Famine will increase until the trend towards capital-intensive food production by the poor for the rich has been replaced by a new kind of labor-intensive, regional, rural autonomy. Beyond a certain level of industrial hubris, nemesis *must* set in, because progress, like the broom of the sorcerer's apprentice, can no longer be turned off.

Defenders of industrial progress are either blind or corrupt if they pretend that they can calculate the price of progress. The torts resulting from nemesis cannot be compensated, calculated, or liquidated. The down-payment for industrial development might seem reasonable but the compound-interest installments on expanding production now accrue in suffering beyond any measure or price. When members of a society are regularly asked to pay an even higher price for industrially defined necessities—in spite of evidence that they are purchasing more suffering with each unit—*Homo economicus,* driven by the pursuit of marginal benefits, turns into *Homo religiosus;* sacrificing himself to industrial ideology. At this point, social behavior begins to resemble that of the drug addict. Expectations become irrational and nightmarish. The self-inflected portion of suffering outweighs the damage done by nature and all the torts inflicted by neighbors. Hubris motivates self-destructive mass behavior. Classical nemesis was the punishment for the rash abuse of privilege. Industrial nemesis is the retribution for dutiful participation in the technical pursuit of dreams unchecked by traditional mythology or rational self-restraint.

War and hunger, pestilence and natural catastrophies, torture and madness remain man's companions, but they are now shaped into a new *Gestalt* by the nemesis that overtakes them. The greater the economic progress of any community, the greater the part played by industrial nemesis in pain, impairment, discrimination, and death. The more intense the reliance on techniques making for dependence, the higher the rate of waste, degradation, and pathogenesis which must be countered by yet other techniques and the larger the work force active in the removal of garbage, in the management of waste, and in the treatment of people made literally redundant by progress.

Reactions to impending disaster still take the form of better educational curricula, more health-maintenance services, or more efficient and less polluting energy transformers, the solutions are still sought in better engineering of industrial systems. The syndrome corresponding to nemesis is recognized, but its etiology is still sought in bad engineering compounded by self-serving management, whether under the control of Wall Street or of The Party. Nemesis is not yet recognized as the materialization of a social answer to a profoundly mistaken ideology, nor is it yet understood as a rampant delusion fostered by the nontechnical, ritual structure of our major industrial institutions. Just as Galileo's contemporaries refused to look through the telescope at Jupiter's moons because they feared that their geocentric worldview would be shaken, so our contemporaries refuse to face nemesis because they feel incapable of putting the autonomous rather than the industrial mode of production at the center of their sociopolitical constructs.

From Inherited Myth to Respectful Procedure

Primitive people have always recognized the power of a symbolic dimension; they have seen themselves as threatened by the tremendous, the awesome, the uncanny. This dimension set boundaries not only to the power of the king and the magician, but also to that of the artisan and the technician. Malinowski claims that only industrial society has allowed the use of available tools to their utmost efficiency; in all other societies, recognizing sacred limits to the use of sword and of plow was a necessary foundation for ethics. Now, after several generations of licentious technology, the finiteness of nature intrudes again upon our consciousness. The limits of the universe are subject to operational probings. Yet at this moment of crisis it would be foolish to found the limits of human actions on some substantive ecological ideology which would modernize the mythic sacredness of nature. The engineering of an eco-religion would be a caricature of traditional hubris. Only a widespread agreement on the procedures through which the autonomy of postindustrial man can be equitably guaranteed will lead to the recognition of the necessary limits to human action.

Common to all ethics is the assumption that the human act is performed within the human condition. Since the various ethical systems assumed, tacitly or explicitly, that this human condition was more or less given, once and for all, the range of human action was narrowly circumscribed.

In our industrialized epoch, however, not only the object but also the very nature of human action is new.[2] Instead of facing gods we confront the blind forces of nature, and instead of facing the dynamic limits of a universe we have now come to know, we act as if these limits did not translate into critical thresholds for human action. Traditionally the categorical imperative could circumscribe and validate action as being truly human. Directly enjoining limits to one's actions, it demanded respect for the equal freedom of others. The loss of a normative "human condition" introduces a newness not only into the human act but also into the human attitude towards the framework in which a person acts. If this action is to remain human after the framework has been deprived of its sacred character, it needs a recognized ethical foundation within a new imperative. This imperative can be summed up only as follows: "Act so that the effect of your action is compatible with the permanence of genuine human life." Very concretely applied, this could mean: "Do not raise radiation levels unless you know that this action will not be visited

---

[2] I have taken this argument, in part, verbatim from Hans Jonas, "Technology and Responsibility: Reflections on the New Task of Ethics," *Social Research* 40 (1972): 31–54.

upon your grandchild." Such an imperative obviously cannot be formulated as long as "genuine human life" is considered an infinitely elastic concept.

Is it possible, without restoring the category of the sacred, to attain the ethics that alone would enable mankind to accept the rigorous discipline of this new imperative? If not, rationalizations could be created for any atrocity: "Why should background radiation not be raised? Our grandchildren will get used to it!" In some instances, fear might help preserve minimal sanity, but only when consequences were fairly imminent. Breeder reactors might not be made operational for fear that they would serve the Mafia for next year's extortions or cause cancer before the operator died. But only the awe of the sacred, with its unqualified veto, has so far proved independent of the computations of mundane self-interest and the solace of uncertainty about remote consequences. This could be reinvoked as an imperative that genuine human life deserves respect both now and in the future. This recourse to the sacred, however, has been blocked in our present crisis. Recourse to faith provides an escape for those who believe, but it cannot be the foundation for an ethical imperative, because faith is either there or not there; if it is absent, the faithful cannot blame the infidel. Recent history has shown that the taboos of traditional cultures are irrelevant in combatting an overextension of industrial production. The taboos were tied to the values of a particular society and its mode of production, and it is precisely those that were irrevocably lost in the process of industrialization.

It is not necessary, probably not feasible, and certainly not desirable to base the limitation of industrial societies on a shared system of substantive beliefs aiming at the common good and enforced by the power of the police. It is possible to find the needed basis for ethical human action without depending on the shared recognition of any ecological dogmatism now in vogue. This alternative to a new ecological religion or ideology is based on an agreement about basic values and on procedural rules.

It can be demonstrated that beyond a certain point in the expansion of industrial production in any major field of value, marginal utilities cease to be equitably distributed and over-all effectiveness begins, simultaneously, to decline. If the industrial mode of production expands beyond a certain stage and continues to impinge on the autonomous mode, increased personal suffering and social dissolution set in. In the interim—between the point of optimal synergy between industrial and autonomous production and the point of maximum tolerable industrial hegemony—political and juridical procedures become necessary to reverse industrial expansion. If these procedures are conducted in a spirit of enlightened self-interest and a desire for survival, and with equitable distribution of social outputs and equitable access to social control, the outcome ought to be a recognition of the carrying capacity of the environment and of the optimal industrial complement to autonomous action needed for the effective pursuit of personal goals. Political procedures oriented to the value of survival in distributive and participatory equity are the only possible rational answer to increasing total management in the name of ecology.

The recovery of personal autonomy will thus be the result of political action reinforcing an ethical awakening. People will want to limit transportation because they want to move efficiently, freely, and with equity; they will limit schooling because they want to share equally the opportunity, time, and motivation to learn *in* rather than *about* the world; people will limit medical therapies because they want to conserve their opportunity and power to heal. They will recognize that only the disciplined limitation of power can provide equitably shared satisfaction.

The recovery of autonomous action will depend, not on new specific goals people share, but on their use of legal and political procedures that permit individuals and groups to resolve conflicts arising from their pursuit of different goals. Better mobility will depend, not on some new kind of transportation system, but on conditions that make personal mobility under personal control more valuable. Better learning opportunities will depend, not on more information about the world better distributed, but on the limitation of capital-intensive production for the sake of interesting working conditions. Better health care will depend, not on some new therapeutic standard, but on the level of willingness and competence to engage in self-care. The recovery of this power depends on the recognition of our present delusions.

The Right to Health

Increasing and irreparable damage accompanies present industrial expansion in all sectors. In medicine this damage appears as iatrogenesis. Iatrogenesis is clinical when pain, sickness, and death result from medical care; it is social when health policies reinforce an industrial organization that generates ill-health; it is cultural and symbolic when medically sponsored behavior and delusions restrict the vital autonomy of people by undermining their competence in growing up, caring for each other, and aging, or when medical intervention cripples personal responses to pain, disability, impairment, anguish, and death.

Most of the remedies now proposed by the social engineers and economists to reduce iatrogenesis include a further increase of medical controls. These so-called remedies generate second-order iatrogenic ills on each of the three critical levels: they render clinical, social, and cultural iatrogenesis self-reinforcing.

The most profound iatrogenic effects of the medical technostructure are a result of those nontechnical functions which support the increasing institutionalization of values. The technical and the nontechnical consequences of institutional medicine coalesce and generate a new kind of suffering: anesthetized, impotent, and solitary survival in a world turned into a hospital ward. Medical nemesis is the experience of people who are largely deprived of any autonomous ability to cope with nature, neighbors, and dreams, and who are technically maintained within environmental, social, and symbolic systems. Medical nemesis cannot be measured, but its experience can be shared. The intensity with which it is experienced will depend on the independence, vitality, and relatedness of each individual.

The perception of nemesis leads to a choice. Either the natural boundaries of human endeavor are estimated, recognized, and translated into politically determined limits, or compulsory survival in a planned and engineered hell is accepted as the alternative to extinction. Until recently the choice between the politics of voluntary poverty and the hell of the systems engineer did not fit into the language of scientists or politicians. Our increasing confrontation with medical nemesis now lends new significance to the alternative: either society must choose the same stringent limits on the kind of goods produced within which all its members may find a guarantee for equal freedom, or society must accept unprecedented hierarchical controls[3] to provide for each member what welfare bureaucracies diagnose as his or her needs.

In several nations the public is now ready for a review of its health-care system. Although there is a serious danger that the forthcoming debate will reinforce the present frustrating medicalization of life. The debate could still become fruitful if attention were focused on medical nemesis, if the recovery of personal responsibility for health care were made the central issue, and if limitations on professional monopolies were made the major goal of legislation. Instead of limiting the resources of doctors and of the institutions that employ them, such legislation would tax medical technology and professional activity until those means that can be handled by laymen were truly available to anyone wanting access to them. In-

---

[3]The Honorable James McRuer, *Ontario Royal Commission Inquiry into Civil Rights* (Toronto: Queen's Printer, 1968, 1969, 1971). On self-governing professions and occupations, see chap. 79. The granting of self-government is a delegation of legislative and judicial functions that can be justified only as a safeguard to public interests.

stead of multiplying the specialists who can grant any one of a variety of sick-roles to people made ill by their work and their life, the new legislation would guarantee the right of people to drop out and to organize for a less destructive way of life in which they have more control of their environment. Instead of restricting access to addictive, dangerous, or useless drugs and procedures, such legislation would shift the full burden of their responsible use onto the sick person and his next of kin. Instead of submitting the physical and mental integrity of citizens to more and more wardens, such legislation would recognize each man's right to define his own health—subject only to limitations imposed by respect for his neighbor's rights. Instead of strengthening the licensing power of specialized peers and government agencies, new legislation would give the public a voice in the election of healers to tax-supported health jobs. Instead of submitting their performance to professional review organizations, new legislation would have them evaluated by the community they serve.

Health as a Virtue

Health designates a process of adaptation. It is not the result of instinct, but of an autonomous yet culturally shaped reaction to socially created reality. It designates the ability to adapt to changing environments, to growing up and to aging, to healing when damaged, to suffering, and to the peaceful expectation of death. Health embraces the future as well, and therefore includes anguish and the inner resources to live with it.

Health designates a process by which each person is responsible, but only in part responsible to others. To be responsible may mean two things. A man is responsible for what he has done, and responsible to another person or group. Only when he feels subjectively responsible or answerable to another person will the consequences of his failure be not criticism, censure, or punishment but regret, remorse, and true repentance.[4] The consequent states of grief and distress are marks of recovery and healing, and are phenomenologically something entirely different from guilt feelings. Health is a task, and as such is not comparable to the physiological balance of beasts. Success in this personal task is in large part the result of the self-awareness, self-discipline, and inner resources by which each person regulates his own daily rhythm and actions, his diet, and his sexual activity. Knowledge encompassing desirable activities, competent performance, the commitment to enhance health in others—these are all learned from the example of peers or elders. These personal activities are shaped and conditioned by the culture in which the individual grows up: patterns of work and leisure, of celebration and sleep, of production and preparation of food and drink, of family relations and politics. Long-tested health patterns that fit a geographic area and a certain technical situation depend to a large extent on long-lasting political autonomy. They depend on the spread of responsibility for healthy habits and for the sociobiological environment. That is, they depend on the dynamic stability of a culture.

The level of public health corresponds to the degree to which the means and responsibility for coping with illness are distributed among the total population. This ability to cope can be enhanced but never replaced by medical intervention or by the hygienic characteristics of the environment. That society which can reduce professional intervention to the minimum will provide the best conditions for health. The greater the potential for autonomous adaptation to self, to others, and to the environment, the less management of adaptation will be needed or tolerated.

A world of optimal and widespread health is obviously a world of minimal and only occasional

---

[4]Alfred Schultz, "Some Equivocations in the Notion of Responsibility," in *Collected Papers,* vol. 2, *Studies in Social Theory* (The Hague: Nijhoff, 1964), pp. 274–6.

medical intervention. Healthy people are those who live in healthy homes on a healthy diet in an environment equally fit for birth, growth, healing, and dying; they are sustained by a culture that enhances the conscious acceptance of limits to population, of aging, of incomplete recovery and ever-imminent death. Healthy people need minimal bureaucratic interference to mate, give birth, share the human condition, and die.

Man's consciously lived fragility, individuality, and relatedness make the experience of pain, of sickness, and of death an integral part of his life. The ability to cope with this trio autonomously is fundamental to his health. As he becomes dependent on the management of his intimacy, he renounces his autonomy and his health *must* decline. The true miracle of modern medicine is diabolical. It consists in making not only individuals but whole populations survive on inhumanly low levels of personal health. Medical nemesis is the negative feedback of a social organization that set out to improve and equalize the opportunity for each man to cope in autonomy and ended by destroying it.

Subject Index
(see also Index of Names)

Index of Names
(see also Subject Index)

ABOUT THE AUTHOR

IVAN ILLICH was born in 1926 in Vienna, Austria, and grew up in Europe. After studies in the natural sciences, he obtained degrees in history, philosophy and theology. In 1950 he came to New York, where he worked for five years as a parish priest in an Irish–Puerto Rican neighborhood. The following five years, he lived in Puerto Rico. Since 1960 he has made his home in Cuernavaca, Mexico. Illich is the author of *Celebration of Awareness* (1969), *Deschooling Society* (1971), *Tools for Conviviality* (1973), and *Energy and Equity* (1974).